SLOW MEDICINE

SLOW MEDICINE

HOPE AND HEALING FOR CHRONIC ILLNESS

MICHAEL FINKELSTEIN, M.D.

wm
WILLIAM MORROW
An Imprint of HarperCollins*Publishers*

A hardcover edition of this book was published under the title *77 Questions for Skillful Living* in 2013 by William Morrow, an imprint of HarperCollins Publishers.

The poem on pages 121–22 is reprinted with the permission of Beyond Words/Atria Publishing Group, a Division of Simon & Schuster, Inc., from *There's a Hole in My Sidewalk: The Romance of Self-Discovery* by Portia Nelson. Copyright © 1993 by Portia Nelson. All rights reserved.

FIRST WILLIAM MORROW PAPERBACK EDITION PUBLISHED 2015.

Designed by Lisa Stokes

The Library of Congress has cataloged the hardcover edition as follows:

Library of Congress Cataloging-in-Publication Data

Finkelstein, Michael (Michael B.)
    77 questions for skillful living : a new path to extraordinary health / Michael Finkelstein, M.D.
        p. cm.
    Includes bibliographical references and index.
    ISBN 978-0-06-222551-1
    1. Health—Miscellanea. 2. Health promotion—Miscellanea. I. Title. II. Title: Seventy-seven questions for skillful living. III. Title: Questions for skillful living.

RA776.F516 2013
613—dc23

2012049851

ISBN 978-0-06-222552-8 (pbk.)

15 16 17 18 19 OV/RRD 10 9 8 7 6 5 4 3 2

To our collective conscious evolution

PHYSICIAN'S PRAYER

Exalted God, before beginning my sacred task to bring healing to Your mortal creatures, I beg You grant me the courage and strength faithfully to execute my duties. Guard me both from the blindness of avarice and the thirst for glory and honor. Endow me with the strength equally to serve the rich and the poor, the good and the wicked, friend and enemy—to simply see in each, a fellow human being in pain. Inspire me with the desire to learn from more learned physicians, for the art of medicine, to which I have dedicated myself, is infinite. Protect me, however, from the scorn and ridicule of those who are older or more respected. Let the truth alone guide me, for any professional compromise can bring only illness and tragedy to Your mortal creatures. O most compassionate and merciful God, strengthen me both in body and soul and implant within me a spirit of wholeness.

—*Moses Maimonides*[1]

CONTENTS

FOREWORD

IN MY FORTY YEARS AS A FAMILY PHYSICIAN, I've yet to see a more practical and comprehensive approach for experiencing optimal health and a fulfilled life than slow medicine. Through this new paradigm, Dr. Michael Finkelstein—a highly respected, board-certified internist—provides you with a fresh perspective on the meaning of *health*. You'll soon learn that health is far more than the absence of illness; it is a state of wholeness and balance of body, mind, and soul. His teaching method is simple yet profound. He's asking you questions that require some reflection to answer. And in that response you'll find *what health means to you*.

The journey you're about to embark on is a life-changing adventure. It is a self-healing process that allows you to safely explore every facet of your life, led by an extraordinary physician, healer, and teacher. Based on what you've learned about yourself, you'll quickly develop the capacity to make healthier, more conscious choices as you transform into a skillful self-caretaker. Your intention and attention will be directed at mastering the art of self-compassion. As you gain greater clarity about the causes of your dis*ease* (physical, mental, emotional, and spiritual)—along with a deeper understanding and appreciation for your gifts, passions, and your life's purpose—health and happiness will flow freely.

Unlike most self-help and medical books on the market, *Slow Medicine* does not suggest that one size fits all. *And that is why it is more useful to you as an individual.* We've been conditioned by a health care system superficially focused on determining what we should weigh or what our BMI should be, based on height and body frame; defining the limits of normal blood pressure, blood sugar, and cholesterol; and recommending how much time we should spend exercising each week, as if we are all the same. Of course, these are all important measures of physical well-being, but the slow medicine prescription of Skillful Living takes you far beyond these standards to a condition of *health marked by greater vitality, peace of mind, an open heart, and an awakened and soothed soul.*

Similarly, conventional medicine excels at treating acute and life-threatening illness and injuries. Yet the high-tech medicine of the West is low-touch and limited, which is not only expensive but regrettably ineffective for curing most chronic conditions, whether it's heart disease, cancer, high blood pressure, arthritis, diabetes, back pain, migraine headaches, sinusitis, or asthma. In fact, the standard of care for the vast majority of these conditions is merely *management*—not true wellness. And we pay for this dearly, not only with dollars but with the pain and suffering that persists unaided.

Approximately 85 percent of our two-trillion-dollar health care expenditures are spent on treating these chronic problems, most of which are preventable and often result from an unhealthy lifestyle. Today's health care industry is a badly broken system, largely because it's become a hugely profitable disease-treatment (some might say "symptom-treatment") *business* with a lot less emphasis on *caring.* Modern medicine is overly concerned with the science to the exclusion of the art of medicine. We deserve something better.

Disenchanted with the quality of care and, for many, the prohibitive expense, Americans are moving away from a dependence on the medical profession for their primary care and are taking more responsibility for their own health. As a result, we've seen a meteoric rise in the practice of *self-care*—learning to eat healthier, exercise more consistently, manage stress more effectively, meditate, and seek greater spirituality in life. Not surprisingly, this trend has been the catalyst for the birth of a new medical specialty: Integrative Holistic Medicine (IHM).

IHM is defined as the art and science of healing that addresses care of the whole person—body, mind, and spirit. The *practice* of IHM is focused on creating optimal health, and treating and preventing chronic dis*ease* by mitigating causes. It's based on the *belief* that unconditional love is life's most powerful healer and that the perceived loss of love is our greatest health risk. This book will help you to write your own unique slow medicine prescription for *loving yourself* in every realm of your life.

IHM has proven to be highly successful in treating myriad chronic conditions. There are currently close to two thousand physicians (M.D.s and D.O.s) in the United States who are board certified by the American Board of Integrative Holistic Medicine, the vast majority of whom are primary care physicians. Michael and I are among this group of pioneers setting a new standard for twenty-first-century health care.

This book will provide you with a wonderful opportunity for practicing this new brand of health care on yourself, combining modern medicine with ancient wisdom, while being guided by a highly skilled primary care physician. Learning to live with skill leads to a state of being *fully alive*. Indeed, that is your answer. My suggestion is that you take your time and delight in the gift that you've given yourself: Indeed, it's time for a dose of *Slow Medicine*.

—*Dr. Rob Ivker, D.O.*

Dr. Ivker is the founder and medical director of Fully Alive Medicine in Boulder, Colorado. The cofounder and former president of the American Board of Integrative Holistic Medicine, he is the author of *Sinus Survival: The Holistic Medical Treatment for Sinusitis* and *Thriving: The Holistic Guide to Optimal Health for Men*.

INTRODUCTION

YOU'VE COME TO THE RIGHT PLACE

Midway along the journey of our life
I woke to find myself in some dark woods,
for I had wandered off from the straight path.

—Dante[1]

WHAT ARE THE CHANCES YOU'VE GOT or will get a chronic medical condition such as diabetes, heart disease, cancer, headaches, arthritis, backache, or stomach trouble? What are the chances you've tried a lot of potential remedies for your condition—a lot of doctors, a lot of pills, a lot of treatments? And what are the chances you're *still* suffering, and find yourself anxious about your health and your future? Speaking as a doctor with a lot of experience, I can tell you the chances are very high. Every day, people just like you arrive at my office looking pained, desperate for relief, and just about hopeless. The fact that you've picked up this book means you're probably a lot like those people. You or someone you love probably suffers from an aggravating health problem that often seems out of control, even though you or they have seen plenty of smart doctors.

There's good news for you. There's no health challenge you face that won't get better with my slow medicine Rx: 77 Questions for

Skillful Living. I'm here to tell you that patients with *all* of the most common health challenges begin to see improvement in their overall health, their specific condition, and their health outlook on the very first day they begin the program outlined in this book.

Whether you're facing a particular health or personal challenge, trying to muddle through the dizzying array of available health information, seeking greater balance in your day-to-day life, or even taking care of a loved one with a health problem, it's my sincerest hope that this book will provide you with needed insights and inspiration. I'm confident that if you take this process seriously, open your mind to an expanded definition of health, complete a comprehensive survey of your condition, and devote the necessary time and energy to answer the 77 Skillful Questions I'm going to present, your health *will* improve. I'm going to tell you about those questions and explain in detail what I mean by "an expanded definition of health" soon, and I think you'll be excited about the prospect.

Meantime, the fact that you've picked up this book encourages me greatly: it means that despite your years of disappointment with the standard of care in our health system, you intuitively understand there *are* answers for even the most persistent and destructive health problems—and these answers lie largely in your own reckoning, in your own hands.

While I make the promise up front that your health can improve, there are a few caveats. I can't promise to give you a Band-Aid solution or some other quick fix. You've tried that before, and I think you know that health just doesn't work that way. I can't promise that every specific health challenge you might have will simply vanish by wishing it away. It won't, and you probably understand why. But I trust that you understand there might be another way to deal with the symptoms you're experiencing and the challenges you face. That's why I wrote this book, and why you're reading it.

I'm not going to water down the message, either. I believe that each one of us has the intelligence, the ability, and the responsibility to make better choices. Again, I promise if you keep your mind open and devote the necessary attention to the whole of your life, your problems will diminish—you'll get healthier. And this form of health will be more achievable, more extensive, more sustainable. It will be, in a word, *extraordinary*.

By contrast, most health books give people messages that they want to hear, packaged in a way that's safe and comfortable and easy: *Lose 30 Pounds in 30 Days! Kick Smoking with Kiwi Juice!* The advice comes sugarcoated and oversimplified. The truth is, extraordinary health requires that we actually face and embrace our challenges, that we dig deep into our lives and look at all the roots and branches. Programs based on simple, formulaic prescriptions often lack this kind of examination, addressing only one specific health issue, such as weight loss or high blood pressure. True, following such advice will sometimes work in the short term, but you know the benefits won't last, because such programs are not designed to be truly integrated into the whole of your life, as a part of meaningful life change.

Also lost in this kind of advice is the real value in our becoming as interested in *learning* from our health challenges as we are in finding quick fixes for them. Finally, such counsel lacks a fundamental honesty: that sometimes, you just have to learn to live with certain conditions; that such a life can be "healthy" and offer infinitely more rewarding prospects than you can imagine.

What else can I promise? I can promise you will finally regain control, starting this very day. By taking the approach that I will outline and guide you through, you will start to see how everything in your life fits together like puzzle pieces to create your overall health picture. This alone will provide a sense of relief. Then, by asking yourself certain key questions about your condition and your life, you'll see where you need to take action, where holes in that puzzle are making a brighter future difficult to discern. You'll be able to formulate a plan that makes complete sense and allows you, step by step, to put the pieces of your life and health back together. Sooner than you think, maybe even immediately, you will begin to feel something you might not have experienced since childhood: a powerful sense of vitality, vigor, serenity—and hope for the future. This might feel unfamiliar at first, maybe even slightly uncomfortable. But you will eventually come to recognize this feeling as extraordinary health, and you'll want to embrace it like a long-lost friend. As a physician, healer, and fellow health traveler, it's my deepest desire to help facilitate that reunion.

It won't always be easy or obvious. I ask you to lend me your trust for a short while as I introduce you to what I call Skillful Questions, which encourage us to think about those aspects of our health and our overall lives that we often neglect—but which have profound consequences on the way we feel. That's what they did for me when I first encountered Dr. Robert Ivker's Wellness Self Test, now called the Fully Alive Questionnaire, the prototype for the Skillful Questions that comprise the formula for this book.[2] The questions and our thoughtful answers gently coach us to live our lives more effectively, more harmoniously with nature and our surroundings, and certainly more healthfully.

To find true health, we must consider an expanded paradigm for health that intelligently—skillfully—integrates science, spirit, and nature. This approach is far-reaching—it goes way beyond simply lowering our weight or blood sugar. But this sensible, "integrative" approach doesn't burn bridges to conventional medicine. Instead, it bridges gaps.

While my definition of health is broader than you're probably used to, I have a pretty simple slow medicine prescription to help you get to that state of health. I call it Skillful Living—an approach that you can develop and learn, just as you might hone the skills of fly-fishing, gourmet cooking, or knitting. This approach is built on four principles:

1. Asking the right questions
2. Identifying the right path
3. Transforming obstacles into opportunities
4. Growing with every turn

Getting healthy starts with asking the right questions. Some of the questions you'll find here are simple and straightforward, and following through on them will seem easy or obvious: I'll ask you if your water intake is adequate and whether you maintain a healthy diet. But as we progress in the program, you might find some of the questions more surprising, and perhaps even a little disconcerting: I'll ask you if you're happy with your sex life and whether you've resolved lingering issues in your relationships with your children and your parents. I will ask you to open your heart and mind to such questions—in some ways to take a leap of faith—and suspend your usual thinking about conventional medicine and the reductionist way it's trained us all to think about the human body and health in general. In my opinion, if you can't do that, you can't really ever get healthy, even if all your "numbers" are good.

I know this process might at first seem daunting. But how daunting is the prospect of continuing to feel the way you've been feeling? To keep running on that hamster wheel of health care until you burn yourself out? I assure you that I know what you're going through: I know the pain, I know the frustration, and I know the despair that attends long-term health challenges when it seems they will never go away. But I also know, from personal experience and from guiding thousands of people like you through this journey, that it doesn't have to be that way. You don't have to feel this way anymore. Sure, as with everything worthwhile in life, you'll have to spend time and energy going beyond conventional medicine. But aren't you worth it? Isn't it time? What do you have to lose?

A NEW DEFINITION OF HEALTH

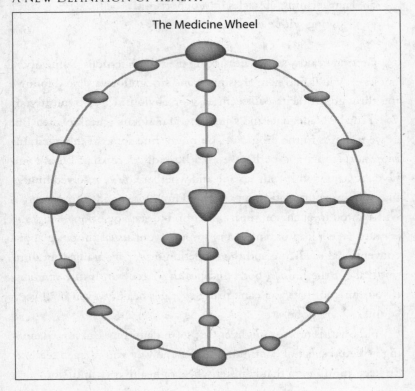

The Medicine Wheel

What do you think is the first thing that comes to mind when you ask the average person to define "health"? Is it as simple as a healthy state of well-being free from disease?

Are you prepared to shift your view and think of health in much broader terms than toned muscles, clear skin, a youthful glow, a low resting heart rate and cholesterol level, or the affirmation of these by well-intentioned physicians? Are you willing to go beyond the limited and limiting definition of conventional medicine into more skillful terrain? I hope so!

You know, it's only a recent phenomenon that we've reduced the idea of "health" to such narrow diagnostic terms. Have you ever seen a traditional Native American medicine wheel? It provides a good example of what I mean by "beyond" conventional medicine. The wheel has four distinct quadrants, representing the physical, mental, emotional, and spiritual realms of human existence. Each of these quadrants works with the others to help one achieve a balanced, harmonious, and healthy life. The archetypal twelve-pointed medicine wheel represents more than just heart, lung, and digestive health, but goes well beyond, taking in the core Native American values of gratitude, respect, speaking, hearing, honoring, service, walking, loving, learning, working, and acceptance. These values in turn form the foundation of integrity (another word for "wholeness"), balance, and happiness on which traditional Native American society operates, and from which we can learn a lot. These Cycles of Truth, as they are often called, clearly show that the concept of "authentic" (healthy) life in Native American society transcends oversimplified definitions of "health" and "medicine" to encompass unity of mind, body, and spirit. It's about living a "skillful" existence in harmony with the universe. That's what I wish for you.

Maybe you think all that's hokey or New Age. That's okay. I don't need you to start dancing around a campfire. I just want you to get healthier. In order to do that, it's important to recognize that "to heal" and "to make whole" are very similar concepts. It's a great tragedy that the modern medical model has abandoned the concept of wholeness, which, to me, is the true meaning of health. I like the word "wholeness," because it implies unity. At times we may be working with specific parts of the body, but we should never lose sight of the whole.

The health we should be looking for is not determined by longevity, wrinkle-free skin, an hourglass figure—or even the complete absence of disease. Look at it this way: Does it really matter that your heart is strong if your relationships with your spouse and children are so awful that you suffer daily agony in your own family? Are you healthy because you're losing weight when all you're eating are some miserably unsatisfying lettuce leaves? How significant is the achievement of finishing the New York City Marathon if you know you're just running away from lingering childhood pain? We must deal with these issues in an integrative way—they're all connected, and they all contribute to our sense of well-being.

Don't be intimidated by the fact that this book is based around seventy-seven questions. It's not a test! And, really, there's just *one* answer we're all after. The 77 Skillful Questions in this book will help reveal our *whole* state of health. They fall into four key categories, all of which work together in creating our overall health:

1. Self
2. Relationships
3. Nature
4. Beyond

How these four dimensions interact is what we experience as health, and as a result, they are the keys to unlocking what ails us— from chronic inflammation to heart disease to psychic pain. I will constantly remind you how the physical self is just a single component of a broader matrix of health. I'll share anecdotes from my practice to expand and reframe your understanding of how these physical, psychological, environmental, and spiritual factors connect to our wellness. Yes, there are physiological symptoms of, say, abdominal distress, and some of those can be eased with physical treatments. But no less important are the other causes of the condition, the underlying sources of the disorder, which often lie well outside the stomach and the intestines—causes such as unhealthy relationships, ignorance of natural cycles, and negative energies.

I'm going to guide you through the list of 77 Skillful Questions that connect all the dots and reveal what's really going on with your overall state of health:

- Whether we have a purpose in life—i.e., how satisfying and fulfilling our work and life missions are
- The quality of our relationships today
- How in tune we are with the rhythms of nature
- How we maintain our connection to life before and after us

But understanding that we're most healthy when we've best integrated all the parts of ourselves does not necessarily translate to success. Once again, we have to ask the right questions to uncover our real current state of health, beginning with the correct definition of "health" itself; we have to answer honestly and completely; and, most important, we have to execute a sensible plan to work on each of those areas, with a specific goal in mind. Although I'd like to get you to think deeply about your health and your life, the plan you undertake will be practical, not academic and theoretical. When we do this, even when we do it gradually, slowly, and incrementally, we begin to experience true health. Here's the kind of health I'm talking about, an integrated paradigm I want you to keep in mind as we proceed:

Health is a natural state of wholeness, marked by the establishment of dynamic balance, encompassing and fully integrating the areas of our mental/emotional, physical, spiritual, social, and environmental condition.

THE 77 SKILLFUL QUESTIONS

How do we get there? My slow medicine prescription is called Skillful Living, a commonsense approach to the practical day-to-day way we conduct our lives. Living skillfully reflects a wiser orientation that will help propel your health forward. It will help you filter all the other advice you receive and test it for its compatibility with your goals, without compromising the integrity of your life along the way.

A foundation of my philosophy is that we should live our lives more skillfully. What does "skillful" mean in this context?

Sure, we all want our headaches and toe fungus to go away—but what if we could make more sense of our lives to boot? What if we could learn to overcome our most pernicious challenges in and out of the health arena? What if we could be healthier and happier at the same time? What if we finally realized how interconnected those two seemingly disparate states are? What if we could make our lives worth living, even when we must experience pain and loss and frustration? What if all our friends and the world were aligned in support of this ideal? It's not just a dream. We can achieve this, if we ask the right questions and follow through. The most important step in Skillful Living is that we learn to ask the best questions that we can of ourselves. Better questions make for better answers. And the first questions in the Skillful Living survey ask us to reflect on the question of health itself: What is health for us, and how can we find it? If health is defined by benchmark numbers—such as the ideal blood sugar and blood pressure—then, sure, we will pursue them. These are often valuable frames of reference, especially if we aim for optimal rather than just acceptable numbers. Yet we'll soon find out that sometimes "normal" numbers often don't make for normal, balanced, or particularly "healthy" lives when we consider life's entirety, inclusive of our true well-being, the feeling state that inhabits our mind all the time and determines the quality of our experience while alive. Again, your level of happiness, balance, peace, and control matter a lot more to your overall health than the difference between a 100/65 and a 130/90 blood pressure reading.

Asking the right questions, and taking an honest look at ourselves, is critical to revealing our current and true state of health in this expanded definition, and to determining the unique ideal we've set for ourselves. In developing the 77 Skillful Questions, I relied heavily on the Wellness Self Test, which was designed by my friend Dr. Robert Ivker and his colleagues at the American Board of Integrative Holistic Medicine for exactly the same purpose as mine. I adopted, adapted, expanded, and fine-tuned these questions, using a number of other influences, including extensive trial and error in my practice; surveying of patients and doctors; collaboration from wise friends and colleagues; and incorporating other traditions, such as Native American and Taoist. What I've come up with is the most extensive and comprehensive list out there.

Simply by asking yourself these questions, you can begin to become more in touch with your own innate intelligence and get reacquainted with your intuitive sense of what you really need. In so doing, you will restore your confidence in your ability to see things clearly, including the best path to actually getting the health you want.

However, to reiterate, the 77 Skillful Questions don't call for us to reject science. They include conventional medicine, then transcend it—making the best use of the science, but placing it into a broader frame of reference. For example, what if I asked you, right now, the following questions:

- Are you aware of and able to safely express anger?
- Do you believe it is possible to change on a fundamental level?
- Are creative activities a part of your work or leisure time?

Would you believe that these things have anything to do with your current and future states of health? What if I told you they're as important as your blood pressure or your weight—in fact, they're so intimately tied up with your physical health that they cannot be extricated from it? I'm sure your doctor has never asked you these kinds of questions before. But I'm equally certain that if he or she did ask—and if you both considered your answers to these questions—he or she would be far better prepared to help you heal yourself of many of your physical problems. And I know that if your doctor helped guide you through a series of questions like these, that process alone would dramatically improve the quality of your health, even without any other treatment.

As we move through all the questions, keep in mind both your current health condition and your health goals and objectives. We'll return to these as our work together progresses. You might find, as our exploration moves forward, that your questions and goals change. My role, as a skillful doctor, is not to simply give you "right" answers, but to help you ask the right questions and learn to find the answers for yourself.

MY MEDICAL A-GAME

I've been asking those questions of myself for a long time. I think I was around seven when my grandmother first said to me, "Michael, you should become a doctor." Perhaps auspiciously, that same year I also failed penmanship—my career path seemed destined! And, as it turned out, growing up I was fascinated with nature and enjoyed studying it, so a career in medicine seemed to suit me. Twenty years later, through equal amounts of determination, focus, and hard work, I fulfilled my ambition of becoming a doctor.

I was already well into a successful medical career when I learned that the word "doctor" actually means "teacher," its origin rooted in the Latin verb *docere,* to teach. This realization was perhaps the first step on the new career path upon which I was about to embark. It caused a critical shift in thinking that's at the core of my health belief system now and forms the basis for this book. Like many doctors, up until that point, I had the feeling that something was missing from my career as a doctor and my mission to help people enjoy better health. For much of the time I practiced medicine, I was haunted by a peculiar sense that I was somehow out of place—that system itself was so limited and limiting that I felt uneasy all the time. I wasn't really *healing* people, and I certainly wasn't helping them heal themselves by the right thoughts and actions. Instead, I saw a revolving door of suffering patients, wrote a lot of prescriptions, dispensed a lot of pills. I had very little time or opportunity to get to know any of my patients the way I wanted to—in a way that would help shed light on their larger lives.

While my patients thanked me a lot, I knew they were as unhappy as I with the sorry state of our health care system. While the United States spends about two trillion dollars on health care annually, Americans by and large find the system complicated, expensive, wasteful, and underperforming.[3] Indeed, 66 percent of those surveyed give the health care system a grade of C or lower.[4] A C! Where I come from, if I brought home a C, I'd be hitting the books until I brought that grade way up. Americans on the whole, of course, are not particularly healthy despite all the money we spend and scientific advances we make—in fact, I'd grade us at about a C minus, if that. I want to deliver, and I want you to receive, A-level medicine—the essence of which, ironically, we can find summarized through a simple nursery school song: *The knee bone is connected to the thigh bone; the thigh bone is connected to the hip bone . . .*

If we're chronically sick, tired, or depressed, we need an examination that includes, but goes beyond, the exact location of our symptoms. That's because everything is inter-dependent—muscles and nerves, bodies and minds, people and planet. Each connecting thread has a domino effect on the other. Toxins in our neighborhood, for example, might cause liver damage, leading to chronic illness that makes us unable to get out of the house or work—leaving us isolated, broke, and as a result, severely depressed. In this scenario, the quick fix of anti-depressants will overlook the root of, and therefore solution for, our depression.

To achieve and sustain optimal health, we need perspective that goes beyond the obvious symptoms. Yes, we need to zoom our lens on the area first calling for attention, but then we must pan our lens to take in the bigger picture, and finally, use our intelligence and intuition to connect all the dots in-between. We need to become aware of each area of our lives and explore how to optimize our wellness, not only within each of these areas—through nutrient-dense foods, a loving partner, artistic expression, and so on—but also through their harmonious *integration*.

We all have the capacity to understand the interconnected web of our health and to channel that domino effect in a positive direction. This individualized process requires exploration and experimentation, patience and perseverance, which takes time but ultimately allows us to cultivate lasting wellness. The best "quick fix" for your health, you see, is not a quick fix at all; rather, it is slow medicine—a methodical, step-by-step process of asking questions that lead to awareness that turns into action that results in extraordinary health. And along the way, as you embark on this journey of discovery, you'll find treasure on the side of the path. Indeed, there's even more waiting for you than the mere relief of symptoms.

Are you ready to begin?

1

UNDERSTANDING YOUR HEALTH: ASKING THE RIGHT QUESTIONS

To find health should be the object of the doctor. Anyone can find disease.

—Andrew T. Still, M.D., Founder of Osteopathy [1]

1. What Brings You Here?

"WHAT BRINGS YOU HERE?" This is the question I use to begin every consultation, so it's the question with which I begin our time together in this book. If you were sitting across from me in my office, we would try to get to the bottom of the following questions: Why have you come to me? Are you suffering from a particular condition or ailment? Are you trying to understand why you're feeling a certain way? Are you frustrated with the contradictory information and limited guidance you've been receiving from others? Have you gotten too much information, and has that confused you about where to begin?

With all that you read and are told by others, do you really understand what it means to be healthy? Unlike most doctors, I am a doctor of slow medicine, meaning I really want to spend time on your questions. They show me where you are on the road to health.

Are you asking good, skillful questions? Think of it this way: you might have the intention to get to New York City from rural Pennsylvania, but by asking for directions to "the big city with all the buildings," you might very well wind up in Philadelphia. Philly's a good town, but it's not where you intended to go. Similarly, if you don't know where you are right now, it will be impossible to find the right road to where you want to go.

The fact is, you probably don't need to think too hard about what's bothering you right now, but you do need to refine your questions in order to reveal the path to true health. So, we start our consultation together with a series of intelligent questions. In general, they can be answered yes or no. This first one, for obvious reasons, is different. As you gain more insight by asking and answering these questions, you'll get a glimpse of a much more optimistic framework for living your life—on a much more interesting journey, I might add. Ultimately, you'll find a more sensible path toward healing.

I've spent a long time walking and studying that path. I'll tell you more about my journey later. For now, I want to get straight to you. Why have you come to me? Like millions of us, you've probably got some health "issues," and some of them might seriously diminish your quality of life. You might suffer from diabetes, hypertension, cancer, arthritis, headaches, ulcers, back pain, or a host of other very common and very unpleasant chronic conditions. You're not alone. According to the Centers for Disease Control and Prevention, more than 133 million Americans (one in every two adults) suffers from at least one chronic illness. The percentage of children and adolescents with a chronic illness has more than quadrupled since the 1960s. And chronic diseases cause seven in ten deaths in the United States each year.[2] You've probably tried a lot of solutions: several doctors, several specialists, several drugs, several "alternative cures," and maybe even several invasive procedures or even surgeries. If you've been suffering for years, you're probably like the vast majority of Americans—a whopping 72 percent—who believe the health care system in America is facing both "crisis and major problems"[3] in part because it can't seem to help you and those other millions.

In any case, if you're dealing daily with chronic conditions, you don't need much in the way of reminders and statistics. What's wrong with this picture? How is it possible that we live in the most technologically advanced period in history, in the richest nation in history, where research, science, and the quest for health and longevity reign supreme—yet so many of us go on suffering needlessly with nasty conditions that are largely within our control? Is it really okay that 16 percent of our country's wealth is spent on medical care—more than any other nation—yet there's precious little evidence that our extra spending makes us healthier?[4] Indeed, we rank only average or below average for health among highly industrialized nations! Why is it okay that so many new drugs were approved by the FDA in the past several years, billions were spent on medical research, doctors got supposedly better and better educations, but the rates of chronic ailments like diabetes and obesity are dramatically rising rather than falling?[5] I'm trying not to sound shrill here, but it's hard. The system is not serving us well, and it's on the brink of collapse.

Meantime, you're still sick, and that's the most important thing. There are several reasons you're sick and why conventional medicine hasn't helped you get well. But I want to focus on a major one that's in your sphere of control: the slow medicine notion that we need to address *all* the aspects of your life, rather than just trying to "fix a broken part," in order to create the best health possible.

2. Are You Free of All Aches, Pains, and Chronic Diseases?

. . . .

THE BIG 8 AND THEIR COMMON CULPRIT

So what does bring you here? Are you free of all aches, pains, ailments, and chronic diseases? This is the first of the yes-or-no questions designed to get you thinking about the bigger picture of health. I hope you're free of all these maladies—but that's not likely.

When we first meet, I encourage each patient to tell me the answer to this question about themselves, their health, and their life. In part, this is to help me understand your history, the particular circumstances of your baseline state of health, and your needs. But it has another, perhaps even more important function: to help you better understand *yourself* and your state of health. Obviously, this particular function is critical in my relationship with you, the reader, because I'm guiding you through a process you're doing at home.

Your health is complex and multifaceted. Symptoms and syndromes are part of a whole web of body and life aspects we'll explore in this book. But let's start at the beginning, on a purely physical (symptom-based) level. Most people first come to me with a concern about a physical problem. The most common presenting complaints fall into one of eight broad categories. Chances are your immediate and initial health concern falls into one of these broad groups, too, some of which overlap:

1. **Chronic pain**. Headaches, migraines, arthritis, backaches, joint pain, muscle pain, neurological pain, menstrual pain, and various other kinds of long-term and debilitating pain

2. **Fatigue**. Lethargy, malaise, sleeplessness, chronic fatigue syndrome, and other low-energy states

3. **Digestive tract issues**. Irritable bowel syndrome, gastroenteritis, colitis, diverticulitis, inflammatory bowel disease, ulcers, and indigestion

4. **Vascular disease**. Heart and circulatory issues along with their frequent partners: obesity, high blood pressure, diabetes, and high cholesterol

5. **Respiratory problems**. Asthma, allergies, frequent bronchitis, emphysema, and chronic obstructive pulmonary disease (COPD)

6. **Mood disturbances**. Depression, anxiety, and other dysthymic conditions

7. **Immune system disorders**. Rheumatoid arthritis, lupus, and other chronic infections and autoimmune syndromes

8. **Cancer**.

3. Do You Understand the Causes of Your Chronic Physical Conditions?

You might have other ailments—and don't worry, I'll address as many as I can throughout this book. But the list above encompasses the main complaints. And this is a very interesting list of symptoms and conditions, from a medical point of view. Can you tell what the common denominator is for essentially all of these?

If you guessed *inflammation,* you're right! It might not be the sole cause, but I can tell you from long experience and solid science there's a good chance that some form of inflammation is at the root of all these physical challenges. It's even implicated in Alzheimer's disease and aging itself.

Inflammation happens to be one of the body's natural protective healing processes. Inflammation is an automatic reaction to an injury or a disease state that precedes it. So a conventional doctor might be satisfied that inflammation in the colon (colitis), for example, has some physical cause, such as a blockage or infection in or around the colon. When they see colitis, they go in search of this cause: What's attacking the colon, causing the inflammation? Notice that their search will focus on the physical cause. In an acute state of inflammation, there often is a physical cause. But the inflammation can persist for a long time without the original insult being present anymore. This is a *chronic* state of inflammation, during which some internal imbalance in the body keeps the inflammation going despite the absence of the original physical insult.

It's also important to note that in many cases of chronic inflammation, some X factor—often outside the involved organ, and maybe even outside the body in some other aspect of the patient's life—supports and maintains the inflammation in the system, settling in the colon, in this example. I'd call this secondary inflammation, but it's inflammation nonetheless.

Either way, when I see colitis as a symptom, I will, of course, like your doctor, look for evidence of injury, underlying disease, infection, and so on—but then I will go *beyond*, using a holistic approach that is helpful for all the inflammatory conditions on the Big 8 list. If you're reading this, it's likely that the primary approach you've experienced in conventional medicine has not done the trick.

Indeed, it's this holistic approach to inflammatory conditions that's really instructive as a model for the way slow medicine works. Inflammation is likely to be at the root of many health problems, but the wisest and best approach for treating it must take into consideration that these conditions will defy straightforward, physical remedies in isolation. The patient needs to work on reducing inflammation with a *comprehensive* plan. In other words, as a rule, "Take two ibuprofen and call me in the morning" is not going to be enough. While that treatment plan might help mask symptoms of acute inflammation, it will fall far short of getting to the bottom of the chronic condition and its causes. If you have colitis, we're going to have to address the inflammatory processes both in your colon *and* in the rest of your life.

Before we get to that, though, let's look more closely at the standard of care in conventional medicine. How do most doctors deal with these kinds of conditions, and why do so many patients feel they're not being helped?

DOCTORS WITH MYOPIA

In my practice, the most common answer to Question 1, "What brings you here?" is: "The doctor I've been seeing really isn't helping me." It's remarkable, but almost every patient says something along those lines. They often add, "I don't think my doctor really *gets* it." Part of the reason for this is that your doctor doesn't believe you *can* change. Dr. Tracy Orleans, a health psychologist at the Fox Chase Cancer Control Center in Philadelphia, found in his research that two out of three physicians were pessimistic about their patients' ability to change. That's perhaps because of poor "compliance" by patients in the past. The doctor tells you to quit smoking and you don't. The doctor tells you to lose weight, yet you "refuse" to change your diet and start moving. Dr. Orleans writes, "This pessimism is the single biggest obstacle to getting physicians to help their patients with their health problems." Yet studies show that if doctors took preventive medicine more seriously, they could *double* the number of patients with better results, like quitting smoking.[6] That's remarkable and disturbing, isn't it?

My doctor isn't really helping me. I don't think he gets it. What you usually mean by that is that your doctor isn't asking you the right questions or guiding you to ask yourself the right questions. Like many frustrated patients, you have an intuitive sense that you need to develop a broader, more comprehensive and holistic treatment plan—but the system doesn't have a lot of room for that. The fact is, you've been trained to be satisfied with the prescription of a pill that might or might not reduce your symptoms temporarily. But your problems come back, and you come back to your doctor time and time again, until you find someone like me or finally figure out that so much of your health is under your control. We'll discuss this dilemma and how to resolve it throughout the book.

MEDICAL EVOLUTION AND REVOLUTION

Pretty early in my career, frustrated with conventional medicine, I stopped feeling anxious about the number of patients in the waiting room, and I engaged the patients in my exam room for as long as I needed to. I asked them about their experiences, their disappointments, and their hopes regarding their health and their health care. I talked to dozens of my colleagues. I read a lot. I launched a personal quest to be the best healer and teacher I could be, and vowed to use whatever tools necessary to get me there, whether or not they fit neatly into the pantheon of conventional Western medicine. I studied and fine-tuned what many health industry vanguards like Dr. Andrew Weil and Deepak Chopra before me had begun.

Soon, I found myself feeling more comfortable as I began to embrace my role as a teacher rather than a mere medical mechanic, as many of my colleagues saw themselves—and as the system regarded us doctors. I stopped concentrating on individual symptoms like stomach pain or infertility, and I began to focus much more on the relationships I developed with my patients and all the ways I could help them think more deeply about the whole of their lives. I began to ask them more and more about their joys and traumas, their childhoods and parenthoods, their vocations and avocations, missions and dreams. I incorporated into my "treatment" plans much of what I had learned by studying various healing philosophies, both ancient and modern, Western, Eastern, and beyond. I felt I had gained a broader perspective on our lives as multifaceted constellations with many stars, all of which together form a living universe—*us*.

Gradually, I began to develop effective techniques to help my patients understand how the numerous and seemingly diverse aspects of their lives—things like the quality of their personal relationships and the passion they feel for their life's purpose—are inextricably tied to their sense of health and, indeed, how well they felt. We did this together, through asking and attempting to answer the right kind of questions about ourselves. When we did this, something stunning and miraculous happened, which had happened less frequently in my years practicing the standard of care: my patients felt better! Empirical evidence proved they actually got healthier. They told me, time and again, that they felt *listened to* and *understood* for the first time in their experience with doctors. They felt like someone really cared—that someone actually "gave a crap," in the language they most frequently used. But their success had a lot more to do with their taking the wheel into their own, skillful hands.

Ultimately, through expanding and honing a series of Skillful Questions about all the aspects of our lives—not just our physical symptoms—I came to understand what many great and influential philosophers and medicine men (both men and women!) did before me: it's all connected. Now, I trained as a scientist. I believe in testing hypotheses and carefully reviewing data. I didn't want to judge the efficacy of the slow medicine methodology just by the happy-looking patients piling up outside my office. This is what I found: for gauging a sense of overall health and well-being, factors that might seem "out there" to the average doctor and patient—such as the extent to which we've found a soul mate—seemed to matter just as much as how well we eat and whether we don't abuse drugs and alcohol. This is at once awesomely revolutionary and totally, intuitively obvious.

In this model of understanding health, your conditions, their causes, and the place they hold in your overall life are all part of one whole *being* worth exploring and treating as such. In other words, just as the body is a dynamic system that must remain in balance to maintain health—the hip bone is connected to the thigh bone, and so on—so, too, is the body just a part of a greater gathering of forces. To achieve real health, the body must work in tandem with the mind, the soul, and the spirit. And that assemblage of all the portions of us that make us *us*, in turn needs to exist in equilibrium with even greater forces beyond ourselves. Our marriages and families. Our careers. Nature and the world around us. Universal cycles and rhythms like that of the moon and the sun. A higher power that many people refer to as God. To uncover the extent to which all these complex systems are functioning smoothly and in harmony, I continued to polish the slow medicine approach, incorporating concepts, insights, ideas, and images I gleaned from my patients, the wisdom of the ages, the best insights of modern medicine, and the counsel of many intelligent and helpful colleagues, whom you can read about in the acknowledgments section of this book.

4. Are You Taking More Medicines Than You Would Like?

AND ONE PILL MAKES YOU SMALL . . .

Maybe you're wondering, Why do we need to redefine health when we've got so many great drugs out there? Couldn't I just find the right pill for my problem? Drugs have their place. I've prescribed them, of course. Some drugs, such as insulin, have literally saved millions of lives. Let's be clear, though. If you lose your pancreatic insulin-making function through trauma, infection, or cancer, you will die. So I'm going to prescribe insulin to type 1 diabetics. But what percentage of all diabetics have type 1, insulin-dependent diabetes? About 5 percent.[7] For everyone else—for literally millions of type 2 diabetics—insulin is overprescribed and overused as a quick fix for the poor lifestyle choices the patient makes, and which, by the way, insulin makes so much more convenient. Here, as elsewhere, the so-called solution is in fact a huge part of the problem, not only ignoring the cause of the initial condition and merely masking its symptoms, but substantively contributing to the problem, as well as causing untold other health problems to boot (because insulin is a growth hormone, it stores fat and contributes to weight gain, making the patient less sensitive to the drug while at the same time increasing his need for the drug). Not to mention what's happening psychologically, which is that so many people get "hooked" on the drug, using it to "chase" bad food choices, or wind up feeling depressed that they're dependent on a drug in the first place. If you take a huge shot of insulin after a dozen doughnuts, your blood sugar will look perfectly normal. The long-term cost of this on the body, on the families of diabetics, and on the health care system is unacceptably high.

It's not just insulin. According to the National Center for Health Statistics, half of all Americans take at least one prescription drug, and over the last ten years, this percentage has risen by 10 percent. The use of two or more drugs has increased by about 30 percent. And the number of people who take five or more drugs has nearly *doubled*—accounting for more than 40 percent of older Americans. There's no doubt we're reliant on pharmacology. One out of five children and nine out of ten older Americans are using at least one prescription drug. In the United States, we spend more than $234 billion a year on medicine—more than double what we spent in 1999.[8] Are we getting better because of all these colorful miracle drugs? Or worse?

I understand that it's possible your condition has progressed to the point where you feel you need medicine just to get through your day. Take our common problem of inflammation. Putting aside for the moment the not insignificant potential side effects and risks (like ulcers, kidney failure, overdose, and dependency), anti-inflammatory medications probably provide you with a measure of temporary relief. If you take steroids for bronchitis, for example, the reduced inflammation in your lungs can help you breath better. If you take a nonsteroidal anti-inflammatory drug (NSAID) for joint pain, you might experience a fleeting reduction in inflammation and pain that can help you cope with daily challenges like work and shopping. But opting for the drug-only solution has four inherent problems:

1. Most drugs prescribed for inflammation only mask symptoms—they don't address the underlying problem. What's causing your inflammation in the first place? Without addressing this question, the problem probably won't get better.

2. The body adapts to such drugs and builds up a tolerance that will eventually mean you'll need more or stronger medications to cope.

3. Relying on drugs with no other plan for overall healing reinforces our broken system of searching for Band-Aids when we need prevention and sustainable lifestyle treatments that incorporate our whole beings.

Even the best drugs come with potentially dire consequences. Just listen to the TV commercials advertising the latest medicine. Have you noticed that the list of potential side effects takes much longer to recite than the list of potential benefits? A well-advertised anti-depressant drug recently listed 22 side effects, including "depression" (yes, as a side-effect of an anti-depression drug), "suicidal thoughts and behaviors" (and you thought depression was bad), "decreases in white blood cells" (your infection-fighting cells), "seizures or convulsions," and "increases in blood sugar levels [hyperglycemia], in some cases serious and associated with coma or death."[9] It's no joke. And that's just if you get the dosages and mixtures right. Fatal medication errors increased *sixfold* in one recent twenty-year period. From 1983 to 2004, more than 200,000 people died from accidental medication mistakes.[10] That's the population of Des Moines, Iowa.

Still, even the most caring and well-intentioned doctors are inclined to prescribe the quick fix of pharmaceuticals or surgery, for conditions that need more thoughtful, individualized, and long-term care. That's because doctors have been trained to be overly reliant on external indicators of illness or wellness, and most are further constrained by the limitations of a profit-driven and largely inefficient health care system. Unfortunately, while quick fixes may temporarily mask symptoms or eliminate the immediate threat, they typically fail to get at the root of an issue, especially in the case of chronic illness. Many health challenges, in fact, stem from an imbalance, and quick fixes often add imbalance, thereby exacerbating the original problem and causing a slew of complications.

Throughout this book, I'll talk about the very effective slow medicine alternatives. Not only does slow medicine have *zero* negative side effects, it's packed with a litany of *positive* side effects as well, and it is the kind of medicine you can practice on yourself—identifying the root cause of your health challenges, then creating a thoughtful, step-by-step, and long-term response to them. I'll guide you every step of the way, and together, we will transform you into your strongest advocate, your own best doctor, and your best friend. You will learn how to bring yourself back into balance and not only resolve your primary complaints, but also to benefit elsewhere in your life, as a natural byproduct of the steps you take.

Paradoxically, if the situation is approached mindfully, illness can serve as a catalyst for a new and improved life. Indeed, getting healthy does not need to be a chore; instead, it can be an adventure.

AN ANTI-INFLAMMATORY LIFE

In the meantime, at the least, I'll recommend working on some ways to reduce your dependence on drug solutions. If we ask the question "What brings you here?" and part of your answer includes "pain" or one of the many other Big 8 conditions based in part on inflammation, then why don't we start with implementing Phase 1 of an anti-inflammatory *lifestyle*—instead of just an anti-inflammatory *drug*? We can begin with the straightforward, physical steps you could take, starting today:

- **Increase anti-inflammatory foods**. The more plant-based your diet is, the less inflamed you will be. A balanced mix of whole fruits, vegetables, whole grains, and legumes provides you with solid nutrition, including all the protein you need and an abundance of antioxidants and phytochemicals that battle free radicals and other inflammatory molecules.

- **Reduce inflammatory foods**. Now that you've added all of these healthy and filling foods, it's easier to consider eliminating some of the inflammatory foods you're probably consuming in excess. These include most animal products, including meat, fowl, fish, and dairy. I understand this might take some getting used to. You don't necessarily have to stop eating all meat, but at least start by making it a side to a main course of plant-based foods. To begin with, try cutting animal products by at least half. Also reduce processed foods, such as food made from flour or milled grains; once metabolized, they quickly become sugar and, in excess, are stored as fat, which contributes significantly to inflammation. Alcohol is also inflammatory and should be limited, as are foods that contain a lot of simple sugar, even if they are natural and whole, such as large quantities of fruit in one sitting. Even diet beverages or foods with artificial sweeteners can be inflammatory. The phosphoric acid in carbonated beverages promotes inflammation by adding acid to your system. The same can be said for excess protein in general, which is another reason why large quantities of animal products are problematic. Then there are foods that you might have a particular sensitivity to, whether you're truly allergic or not. In either case, your immune system reacts to some element in these foods, producing damaging free radicals and other inflammatory molecules. Common foods that do this are wheat, dairy, soy, nuts, and chocolate. If you continue to consume the foods to which you are sensitive, in a way you're saying "I want to be in pain," which I know is not really true. You just need better information and better guidance to see how important all this is. The fact is, you can't expect to avoid inflammatory symptoms like pain if you keep putting into your body the things that cause painful inflammation.

• **Start moving more and get outside**. Stagnation is a setup for inflammation. To the extent that you can, get moving to increase circulation and improve your body's ability to release accumulated toxins, work your joints and muscles, lower blood sugar and blood pressure, lose weight, increase peace and balance, and decrease pain and inflammation overall. You don't have to run marathons, but you probably have to do more than you're doing. Haven't you ever wondered why so many of those "tough old birds" of yesteryear managed to live into old age even though they smoked, drank, caroused, and ate a pound of eggs, butter, and bacon every morning? Just look at your couch for an answer. Those people got outside and moved—they were in touch with nature. Most of them were gardeners in one way or another. They lived more connected to the earth in some meaningful way.

• **Get enough water and sleep**. Proper hydration and adequate sleep allow our body's physiological process on a cellular level to work optimally, and ultimately are both necessary to reduce inflammation. Addressing dehydration and sleep deprivation alone might be the single most important step toward the health that has been eluding you.

• **Unload your toxins**. Think about toxins (such as lead, mercury, pesticides) in your home, workplace, and greater environment. Are you exercising too strenuously and producing even more free radicals? Are the bacteria that live in your gut helping you or hurting you? The fact is, we need to "empty the garbage" now and then. While our body does have natural mechanisms to do this, given all that we are exposed to—in the food we eat, the air we breathe, and the water we drink, not to mention the other chemicals that we come in contact with every day—we need to pay special attention to this matter. Clearly, it helps to avoid toxins to begin with, but there are ways to help your body release them once they wind up inside of you. All of the measures mentioned above will help you here. And there are others that you might consider, such as cleansing juices and select periods of fasting.

These steps will all make a very good start, and they will certainly make a dent—often a big one—in the most common health challenges. A random, destructive diet and a couch-potato lifestyle are some of the main causes of inflammation in the body, which in turn contributes substantially to most major health problems, with diabetes and heart issues at the top of the Big 8 list.

But an anti-inflammatory life goes deeper than diet and physical activity. Chances are, when I ask the question "What brings you here?" and your answer reveals an underlying inflammatory condition, a few follow-up questions will reveal some deeper issues. What's going on in your life? Your marriage? Your job? Your school? Your plans for the future? Well, *now* we often discover some rather inflammatory situations worth investigating. Are you fighting tooth and nail with your kids? Are you in the middle of an acrimonious divorce? Are you stressed about money? Do you work in a hostile environment? Are you getting sued? Are your parents ratcheting up the pressure on you? Are you trying—and trying and trying—to get pregnant? Doesn't it make sense that if you began to work on those deeper "inflammatory" and "painful" challenges, the physical manifestations of the inflammation and pain might begin to abate? If it doesn't make sense, I wish you and the medical establishment would humor me and try it. Try working on even one of those situations that's ostensibly outside the realm of your physical health, and see if it doesn't improve your physical health, too, and soon. I can tell you I've done this in my own life, read hundreds of studies that back it up, and seen thousands of my own patients prove it. It might not be a panacea, but it's a hell of a lot more beneficial than popping pills every four hours.

I'm relieved to find that many doctors *are* slowly coming to believe that it is these "outside" issues that are the root of most common ailments. That's especially true of inflammatory conditions. Let's take one of the most common, persistent, and incapacitating conditions: back pain. Dr. John Sarno, professor of clinical rehabilitation medicine at the New York University School of Medicine, has studied back pain for decades and has treated celebrities like Howard Stern, Anne Bancroft, and John Stossel, who've all praised his work. He argues:

> Neck, shoulder, and back pain are not a mechanical problem to be cured by mechanical means. It has to do with people's feelings, their personalities and the vicissitudes of life. Above all, back pain is a reflection of temperament, which is undoubtedly why back pain is so common. Americans are a nation of doers and workers. We take life seriously and responsibly. As our lives become more complex, we generate more and more tension. This is the basis for most back pain.[11]

Sarno believes the same goes for gastrointestinal troubles, skin disorders, and a number of other common inflammatory conditions, and I agree. So let's take this idea even further. Let's say you're totally committed to doing everything in your power to create a life that's as free as possible from inflammatory situations. Your goal is to free yourself of back pain and the rest of the Big 8 by reducing inflammation across all aspects of your life. Here's what you could do for a Phase 2 of the anti-inflammatory lifestyle:

- **Avoid arguing**. Find other ways to release the energy (talking it out, mediation, forgiveness, leaving unsalvageable relationships and hostile jobs, turning the other cheek, getting couples counseling, etc.).

- **Avoid seething**. Practice ways to let go of inner pain and turmoil (from loss, from the perceived hurts of others, from regret, and so on). Therapy often works. Faith. Meditation. The help of a spiritual adviser. Walking and other physical activity. Pets. Volunteering. Sewing, tinkering, gardening, or any other benign and unstrenuous physical activity.

- **Try to resolve ongoing relationship/work problems**. Make a plan to tackle the parts of your life that cause you the most *aggravation* (another word for *inflammation*). If you experience peace and harmony in your everyday life, your body will respond in kind. You won't find perfect solutions, so don't even try. You can't *control* your toddler, your teenager, your boss, that talk-show host of the "other" party, or anyone else for that matter. All you can control is your reactions to them. Don't let others "inflame" your rage, regret, or fear.

- **Seek peace**. Find a peaceful place to meditate or relax
regularly. Listen to music and watch movies that bring you
joy and a sense of calm and serenity. Go out into nature and
listen to the birds. At least watch the fish in your fish tank.
Play with your dog or cat more often. Find regular relief
from work, family, money, and other potential stressors. If
you have to, carve out time and earmark energy for peace-
seeking activities like gentle hiking, watching the sun set,
and sex with someone you love.

- **Avoid inflammatory media**. Consciously avoid
aggravating and incendiary movies and music. This is tough
nowadays. Practice a news embargo at least one day a week.
Bad news and violent films and lyrics provide fuel to the fire
of an already inflamed body.

All these suggestions might fall under the more familiar tent of
"reducing stress." As you know, stress is complicated, but at its core, it
raises blood levels of hormones like cortisol, which are likely agents of
inflammation and therefore of all the Big 8 conditions—including certain kinds of cancer—that we associate with inflammation. I posit that
if you start seriously practicing both phases of the anti-inflammatory
lifestyle plan, you'll get some relief from your condition in as little as
a week.

Perhaps you're skeptical that following this plan could improve your
long-term chronic ailment. Can you at least see that you would feel
much better if you made even moderate improvements in these areas
of your life? If you can't see that yet, stick with me, and I'll go into far
more detail later. Suffice to say here that the answer to Question 3—Do
you understand the causes of your chronic physical conditions?—should
lead you to investigate both physiological causes and what we might

loosely call "metaphysical" contributors—the things in the rest of your life that tend to resonate in your physical body.

5. Do You Feel a Strong Sense of Purpose in Life?

SOMETHING TO LIVE FOR

This is a big question, obviously, to which I've been alluding throughout the introduction and this first chapter. It comes down to a very simple principle, however: What do you have to live for? What would you *use* your good health for if it was returned to you? If you're feeling unconnected to the world around you; if you're floating through jobs, relationships, and homes; if you still don't know what you want to do with your life or why you're even here on Earth, then it's going to be a tough task to maximize your health and well-being. Ask yourself, Who am I? What's my purpose? Who and what do I value in this life—and why? These are meaningful, powerful questions that are bound to bring up strong emotions. Believe it or not, the vast majority of us in modern Western culture never ask such questions, much less attempt to answer them. This is paradoxical, considering many of us can afford the luxury of such introspection.

In short, most of us now have the ability—the time, the expertise, the resources—to organize our lives around a quest for extraordinary health that incorporates a sense of purpose. Extraordinary health is the achievement of a state of wholeness, living a good life in a state of awareness and harmony with those around us and with the greater universe. Ultimately, health is more than just living well, but is marked by peace and tranquillity throughout your life. To be in this state requires the cultivation of mindfulness; identifying and following your passions and purpose; and the recognition of, and ability to express, your essential authentic self. Yes, it's true that many (if not most) of the world's population still seems bound by desperate imperatives like staying alive and subsisting, preventing them from fully exploring such an ideal. But is that true in your life? Can you not afford to take care of yourself? Can you not find the time, the energy, or the tools you need to live skillfully—for as long as possible, in the best health possible, with the best attitude about your health? I think you probably can. And if you truly can't, it would obviously be essential for you first to work diligently on those real obstacles to your achieving health.

However, as a wise early goal, regardless of your relative freedom to expand your health, it's good to think about your purpose in life. For example, at this point in my life, I have come to realize that it's my life's purpose to join and guide others in their quest, and help them achieve the health and happiness they seek. That's why I find it so distressing to see people wandering aimlessly, living without clarity and a higher purpose, and suffering needless physical and psychic pain. The direction of our lives is not predetermined, but when we walk the path into the unknown with purpose and intention, we can grow at every turn. I think you probably get this idea. Thirty million of you read Rick Warren's *The Purpose Driven Life,*[12] which has been credited with stopping crimes and saving lives.[13]

So what's your purpose? I've heard others answer in the following ways, in case you're looking for ideas:

- To experience life fearlessly to its fullest, in all its iterations
- To raise a family I can be proud of
- To contribute meaningfully to the field of poetry and literature
- To serve God
- To never stop learning

- To live up to the gift of my consciousness and the blessing of my senses
- To see as much of the world as possible before I die
- To educate children
- To experience joy, dancing, singing, and bliss as much as possible

You might notice from this list that one's purpose can take two forms: what spiritual teacher Eckhart Tolle calls an "outer purpose," and a corresponding "inner purpose."[14] An outer purpose is what you *do* ("My purpose is to dance professionally in the vanguard of new African American choreography"). From the point of view of your health, this is central. Indeed, as Rick Foster, Greg Hicks, and Jen Seda write in their book *Choosing Brilliant Health,* "You must make central to your life the things you love by acting on them."[15] Health researchers Foster and Hicks conducted years of study on how we find and maintain happiness and good health. One of their central conclusions is that when we go out of our way to engage in activities that uplift and stimulate us emotionally, we get happier. That makes intuitive sense. But they also cite colleagues' studies to prove that "doing what we love increases our satisfaction levels, which correlates strongly with greater longevity."[16]

Think back to your symptoms again. Not too long ago, my nineteen-year-old son, Malcolm, was suffering from a series of sore throats. In my mind, the pressure of final exams during the spring of his freshman year at a competitive college was affecting his immune system and causing inflammation, which settled into a vulnerable area—the throat. It wasn't really important to me whether his sore throats were infectious or not. I knew that he'd recover when his exams were over. But to my surprise, he got better sooner. Why? Because his favorite band, Phish, had just announced its summer tour schedule, and he and some friends made plans to attend an epic six shows in a three-week span. A miracle Phish cure? No. Just a reflection of the healing power of passion. My son's outer purpose was his commitment as a fan to this talented group of musicians. Their music made him happy, made him dance, made his spirit rise—and made him healthier. This has been going on since long before Phish and the Grateful Dead and even the lyre was heard over the hills, all the way back to drum circles and catgut strings that mimic the rhythms of nature.

The inner purpose is different and quite a bit deeper, although it's helpful for it to be aligned with the outer purpose. While Tolle insists that we should all have the same exact inner purpose—to "awaken" and share that awakening with others—I think there's a lot more room for individual development in this area. I believe you should think of your inner purpose not so much in terms of what you *do* (teach, sing, travel, raise kids) but rather in who you *are,* which can extend past the apparent limitations of "teacher," "singer," "traveler," or "parent," if you consider those designations creatively, into something more sublime and perhaps harder to put your finger on at first. It's the thing that makes you *you,* the thing at your core that makes your life worth living, preserving, protecting, and celebrating.

THE HEALING EFFECTS OF PURPOSE

The Japanese have a word for this sense of purpose, which loosely translates to "something to live for": *ikigai*. It's a very old tradition, with some very new science to back up its efficacy for health. In three recent Japanese studies, people with *ikigai* fared better—in some cases much better—than their counterparts without *ikigai* when it came to surviving heart attacks and strokes.[17] You've all heard stories of people who lost their life mates, got sick, and just "gave up" or "willed themselves to die." It really happens; I've seen it many times. But it's proof that you can also *will yourself to live*. It's obviously much, much easier to find your *ikigai* when you believe in your heart that you have something to live for.

Do you think you're too old to develop a life purpose? It's never too late! Finding a purpose is, in fact, not typically the province of the young. But it can help you live a longer and happier life, even when you adopt it late in life. Research conducted by *Ageing International* synthesized more than seventy prior studies on the effects of a purpose-driven life on the body, and found that a personal sense of purpose in life led to better long-term health through middle age and into old age. A lack of purpose was found to be associated with boredom, hopelessness, depression, and the loss of the will to live. More than half of individuals who have a sense of purpose in life have above-average health.[18] It works the other way around, too. Another recent study found that the risk for Alzheimer's disease in the elderly increased when the patients did not have a strong sense of purpose. Those who had a strong sense of purpose were twice as likely to remain free of the disease than those with a low sense of purpose. The results suggest that deriving meaning from life's experiences, and having a goal-oriented mind-set, substantially reduces the rate of cognitive decline in old age.[19] Other studies back up these findings relative to Alzheimer's and related conditions.[20]

This sense of purpose can lower the risk of ailments as banal as the common cold and as brutal as the most aggressive forms of cancer.[21] Dr. Martin Seligman, a pioneer in the study of health and happiness, reviewed eighty-three studies on the effects of pessimism and optimism on mortality from all causes, mortality from cardiovascular disease, immune function, and cancer, and found statistically robust results. He looked at eighteen studies on cancer, including a Women's Health Initiative Study involving 97,252 patients, and concluded that, controlling for other risk factors for cancer, negative mental states like pessimism and hostility are significant predictors of cancer.[22] Bottom line: optimistic patients, including those who have a strong sense of purpose, fare better.[23]

DISCERNING PURPOSE: SOME KEY POINTS

In your quest to divine and develop your own, unique life purpose, keep a few things in mind. You should write your purpose down and solidify it. Keep it short. If you can get it to one or two sentences, great. If you can further distill it to one or two words, even better. It helps, too, to think in images and metaphors. Bring your written purpose out once in a while to tweak or to remind yourself what you're all about when you're feeling lost, misdirected, or kicked around, Nixon-style, by life. Below are some features an ideal purpose would comprise, with some examples of others' purposes to stir your creativity. Your purpose should be:

- *Consistent* **with your values, morals, and ethics**. It's the essence of who you are and what you do; it's the attribute of which you're proudest; it reflects your core beliefs. It's honest and true to *you* and only you. You've chosen it of your own free will. It's how you want others to think about you; what you want them to say about you at your funeral, or to carve on your tombstone along with your name.

    The piper: "My purpose is to find joy and share joy for myself and others through music, whether from my instrument, my voice, or the rhythms and harmonies of the universe."

• ***True* to universally embraced principles**. It isn't incompatible with our shared sense of right and wrong (i.e., it doesn't infringe on the rights of others); it doesn't upend the natural and intuitively "right" balance of values, by placing, for example, a selfish value like greed above a generous one like altruism.

> *The scholar: "My purpose is to learn wherever, whenever, however, and from whomever I can; to always find opportunities for growth and development of my mind through sharing the wisdom of others and the earth, and to pass on what I've learned to others through my writings and teachings without ever succumbing to didacticism."*

• ***Satisfying* and bliss-producing**. It really gets your juices flowing. It makes you happy to think about it, plan it, learn it, do it, teach it, dream about it, and remember it after it's done. If it's the last thing you're thinking, believing, or doing when you die, it'll be, as the Native Americans say, a good day to die.

> *The healer: "My purpose is to learn and practice natural, holistic ways to heal my body and my psyche, then share them with others through the confluence of medicine and spirituality, wherever I'm needed most, and to ensure I take proper care of myself so I can be there to help heal others for as long as possible."*

• ***Varied* enough to hedge against boredom**. It has sufficient variety to keep you on your toes; to keep teaching you new things; to prick up your creative ears; to sustain you during dark times; to encompass your multiple interests, talents, and beliefs.

> *The leader:* "*My purpose is to seek and carry out various ways to bring my community and other communities together in pursuit of peace and positive change that raises the least among us to the highest.*"

• *Resonant* **throughout all facets of your life**. It reflects both what you *do* and who you *are*; it provides a metaphor for the whole way you live your life and interact with others and the environment.

> *The warrior:* "*My purpose is to stand up and fight for justice and fairness wherever it needs an advocate, and to do what's necessary to uphold those principles, especially for those who cannot fight for themselves.*"

• *Meaningful,* **contributory, and legacy-building.** It's important enough in the grand scheme of things to *matter* beyond selfish and transitory desires. It—*you*—will leave a positive legacy long after you're gone, either on individuals, society, or the world as a whole.

> *The philosopher:* "*My purpose is to strive to use my mind and encourage others to use their mental faculties to think deeply about the betterment of our collective, human future, and to execute courses of action to promote wise, sustaining principles.*"

• **Healthful**. It works in accord with your good health and the good health of others; it doesn't flout the natural laws of health by endorsing dangerous or irresponsible behavior. Its practice promotes longevity, vitality, and strength.

> *The ecologist: "My purpose is to do my part and beyond to respect, uphold, and help restore the natural environment around me, including all nonhuman creatures, and to do whatever I can to leave the world in the same or better shape than it was before I entered it."*

This exercise should not be stressful—"Oh my God, what the hell am I doing with my life? I have to find a purpose by eight thirty!"— but rather meditative, contemplative, and restorative. It will probably take some time, and it might require some counsel from people you trust and love. It's amazing how quickly your loved ones can identify what *they* think you're all about, even when you have no idea, and it's amazing how close they get sometimes to what you believe but haven't yet articulated. One of my patients, for example, asked her husband what he thought her purpose was. He said, "Look around!" All over their kitchen were the six dogs they'd recently rescued from a hurricane. "Oh, yeah," she said.

A note: if you're experiencing a serious depression, it can be very painful and very difficult to contemplate, no less articulate, a life purpose. Which comes first here, the chicken or the egg? Are you depressed because you're purposeless—or purposeless because you're depressed? These are questions that get to the very heart of integrative medicine, though I don't think the answer per se particularly matters. What matters is restoring balance and achieving health in the larger context we've been discussing. If you're suffering, know that you *do* have a purpose underneath the pain. I want you to keep reading.

6. Do You Believe It's Posssible to Achieve Genuine, Extraordinary Health?

. . . .

HOW GOOD CAN YOUR HEALTH GET?

If I asked you whether you thought you could ever be truly healthy, there's a good possibility that your knee-jerk response would be "No way. I'm too sick. I'm too fat. I'm hurting too much. My genetics work against me. It's too late." While some of these details might be true, your opinion about their implication is a reflection of what you have been taught and the society in which you live: your conclusions might still be false.

So as you embark on this journey, I urge you to look in the mirror and understand the basis for your current belief system. You might realize that the things you have until now accepted as truth are not absolute, but full of gray areas. In fact, every day we see new ideas, experiences, arguments, and studies challenging even centuries-old beliefs and assumptions. Recently, the very foundations of Christianity were shaken by the discovery of the Book of Allogenes, which scholars now recognize as the only known surviving copy of the Gospel of Judas. Judas! Now there's an alternate perspective on long-accepted "truth." In the field of medicine, which generates so much of the "expert advice" about health, new information and discoveries show us that some of the most time-honored medical practices are simply off the mark.

Remember, the truth, as we have come to know it, can change at any moment, and just might shake our foundation to the core. Therefore, modesty and humility are a necessary part of this new awareness. It's critical to accept and embrace the idea that there might be another way of looking at things. The good news is that even if you've been told you'll never get healthy, you can.

To live skillfully, you might need to shift perspective and alter your course. For some, this could entail nothing more than going to bed an hour earlier. Others might discover that a major shift is in order, such as switching careers or reassessing a marriage. You know now that adopting a new framework for living is not strictly about our physical bodies—avoiding disease or losing weight, looking better and simply living longer—but using personal challenges and obstacles to help find the path to a richer, more authentic existence.

I want you to stop reading at this point and just reflect. Think about the possibilities that are out there for you, health-wise. Believe—really believe and incorporate that belief into your daily thinking process—that you can, that you will, achieve genuine, brilliant health. It may not have worked *yet,* I know. But why not? Because you've probably been going about it the wrong way, thanks to decades of conditioning. There's an old adage, popular in recovery programs, and attributed variously to two of the smartest guys of the past few hundred years, Ben Franklin and Albert Einstein: Doing the same thing again and again and expecting different results is the very definition of insanity.

Stick with this. Start the next chapter with verve and excitement about the new life you can make for yourself, about the extraordinary health that awaits you on the sane side of the street.

Throughout this book, I'm going to offer you some "bonus materials." These will take two forms. The first will be further, practical exercises (but I'm a doctor, so I'm going to call them "prescriptions" instead) designed to get you thinking and moving forward. They will require some action on your part. Please set aside some time in your life to really give these Practical Prescriptions the time and energy they demand. You won't regret it. The second will be bonus questions for further reflection, which I hope you will endeavor to answer for yourself; these are largely self-explanatory.

PRACTICAL PRESCRIPTION 1:
WHAT ARE MY SYMPTOMS OF HEALTH?

Most of us are so habituated to looking for disease that we rarely pay
attention to the health we already possess. We live in a culture where
the complaint is king—where we expect things to be a certain way
and where we have a meltdown or simply give up when they are not.
What might our lives be like if we "celebrate instead of complain,"
in the words of motivational speaker Donna Hartley, who survived
a fatal plane crash, stage III melanoma skin cancer, and open-heart
surgery?

Indeed, there are few experiences more humbling than speaking
with young and wounded soldiers recently back from war. They tend
to define "health" not in clinical, symptom-based terms but rather in
terms of spirit, courage, inner strength, conviction, hope, problem-
solving ability, proactivity, and camaraderie. While they have endured
loss, they are vividly aware that they could have lost so much more. As
a result, they live in appreciation of what they *do* have.

When struggling with our health challenges, it is helpful to learn
about others who have transcended their own limitations. From professional dancers without legs, who move with wheelchairs and pros-
thetics more gracefully than most of us use our feet, to health and
wellness leaders who thrive despite their own "diseases," examples
abound. What mindset empowers these individuals to transcend their
limitations, and how can we adopt this mindset, to shift from surviving to thriving?

So this first Practical Prescription asks you to turn the complaint
habit on its head. Ask yourself: What's working about my health?
Look for *symptoms of well-being.* Frame these questions in the positive.
Write them down. I encourage you to come back and add to your list
as you progress through this book. As you become more skilled at

finding health, your list should get longer, and the items more indicative of expanding health. The following are just examples, not benchmarks to strive for. Your health is your own. Give yourself credit for any health achievement, no matter how small you think it is, because it's all relative. And don't forget that extraordinary health extends well beyond the physical:

- I can play catch with my dog for ten minutes before getting winded
- I can pick up my granddaughter
- I can breathe and appreciate the scent of my garden
- I can dance to the first three tracks on the new Lady Gaga album
- I can get up and down the stairs
- I can appreciate the beautiful scenery
- I can hike all day if it's flat ground
- I can shovel my neighbor's driveway
- I can feel grace and blessings when I look at my family
- I can bowl two games in a row
- I can use all four of my limbs to get through my day
- I can finish a marathon in eight hours
- I can be grateful for my wonderful career as a nurse
- I can wheel myself to the store without my arms getting tired
- I can think, pray, believe, hope, remember, wonder, and plot my future

QUESTIONS FOR FURTHER REFLECTION

7. Do You See an Alignment Between Your Personal and Professional Goals?

8. Does Your Job Use All of Your Greatest Talents, and Is It Enjoyable and Fulfilling?

It's simple: The more you get to do what you love, the less it feels like a job, and the more it feels like a healthy, rewarding, and balanced life. We spend so many hours either at work or thinking about our career that it's ideal if we don't compartmentalize it, but rather integrate it into our overall health plan.

2

AWAKENING YOUR SEVEN SENSES: REGAINING TRUST IN YOURSELF

Through seven figures come sensations for a man; there is hearing for sounds, sight for the visible, nostril for smell, tongue for pleasant or unpleasant tastes, mouth for speech, body for touch. . . . Through these come knowledge or lack of it.

—Hippocrates[1]

I'VE BEEN A DOCTOR for more than twenty-five years, following four intense years in medical school and another four grueling years of residency training at one of New York City's leading hospitals. But if you came for a consultation with me today, you wouldn't find me in a white jacket in a hospital or medical center. Instead, you would drive up a little dirt road in the village of Bedford, New York, and park outside a beautiful old barn, with a green lawn, a gurgling brook, a vegetable garden, and beehives. It's very likely that Stanley or Stella, our resident peacock and peahen, would come over to say hello. They're part of a menagerie of rescued animals that graze in the pastures here. Welcome to SunRaven: The Home of Slow Medicine—

my clinic, my home, and the space I've created to hold and express the intention that individuals and our society as a whole will learn and move forward in their evolution, not merely to rid themselves of ailments, but to achieve a state of peace, tranquillity, harmony, and balance—the essence of true, lasting, extraordinary health.

When you step into my office, I offer you something I believe is worth more than any drug prescription or typical treatment regimen: I help you to learn to help yourself. Early on, I try to start empowering you. I show you that, while a good doctor is valuable, you already possess the more important tools to find the answers for yourself. At the foundation of this philosophy is the profound belief that on some level, you *know* a lot more than you might be consciously aware of on a day-to-day basis. In fact, in a weird paradox occasioned by our information age, our overdependence on the "knowledge" of medical authorities often obscures the deeper knowledge that exists within us. Our five physical senses are naturally attuned to our health. Most of us understand that much. But we need to retrain ourselves to tap into our sixth sense, our intuition, as well. And, going further, I'll assert that we must hone our seventh sense, too—our *common* sense. This chapter is about using all our tools. I am encouraging you to literally "come to your senses."

WESTERN MEDICINE AND WESTERN EXCESS

It's my life mission to help you go beyond conventional medicine to your best, most extraordinary health. To be clear, though, never do I dismiss the achievements of modern medicine. First of all, I'm a skilled clinician, classically trained in one of the finest medical schools. I'm proud of what my profession has accomplished, and I still use my training every day. I don't discredit the many milestones of conventional medicine, nor do I undercut the critical role that my trained and dedicated professional colleagues play in saving lives every day. But if you think about it, we doctors play our A-game only when it comes to acute conditions. If a patient comes into an ER with a compound tibula-fibula fracture, we really rock and roll. We can diagnose, treat, palliate, prevent infection, and generally heal this kind of traumatic injury very well and fairly quickly in the grand scheme of things (especially when you consider that in the not-so-distant past, a broken leg was a possible death sentence). We've come a long way since bloodletting and bone setting were state of the art.

But guess what? In the modern world—in the West, especially— the vast majority of our medical problems are not acute. Proportion- ally, we encounter far more chronic (long-term, debilitating) medical conditions, like high blood sugar and obesity, than we see acute (emer- gent, traumatic) problems like lacerations and infections. And the funny thing is, many acute problems, such as heart attacks and strokes, are very often preventable emergencies that occur almost inevitably as the last stage of poorly managed chronic problems. Meaning, if we treated the chronic conditions properly, we'd have even fewer acute emergencies.

So, first of all, if you have a burst appendix, there's a screwdriver jammed in your thigh, or your eye has popped out of its socket, I highly recommend the standard of care in Western medicine. You can't do much better. But if you're suffering from a more chronic prob- lem, one of those common but exasperating concerns that constitute the great majority of our health challenges—problems like migraines, PMS, joint pain, psoriasis, and the other Big 8 I outlined on pages 18–19—I suggest you look at the "success" rates for the most modern "treatments." The very definition of a chronic condition includes the notion that it does not respond well to quick fixes. It's clear we need to reconsider the way we handle such chronic health problems, which account for the bulk of the "patient load" that is straining our system and slowly killing us and our kin.

The good news here is that over those chronic issues, as frustrating as they are, we can exercise a huge amount of control through slow medicine. In many ways, as unpleasant as it might be to hear this, we got ourselves into our messes—and we can get ourselves out.

Think about it: Can we blame doctors and Western medicine for the failure rates in preventing and curing chronic illnesses? Partly. It's obvious their message is not getting across properly, or rates of chronic diseases would not be rising so precipitously. On the one hand, these problems are simple. If you eat too much and move too little, you gain weight. If you gain too much weight, you're likely to develop a group of other problems—the "metabolic syndrome"—and one or more of these problems, left unchecked, will ultimately put you in the ground. The condition, reframed in this way, is obviously preventable. Eat less junk. Move around more. Problem solved.

It sounds like I'm being facetious, but it's true. Most of the solutions to our most common chronic conditions are just that obvious and just that easy, technically, to solve. Your senses alone, including your intuition and common sense, already have the answers to your problem. In fact, to a great extent, our most pernicious and debilitating chronic ailments (like type 2 diabetes and obesity) are almost entirely within our own control. Weird, isn't it? As a culture, we get smarter every day. We're very proud of our intelligence. We have access to more information than ever before. We spend billions on self-help. We venerate and slaver over the latest diet and health fads. So why don't we get better? Is that our doctors' fault?

We clearly have a cultural problem. The qualities that helped catapult the West into glorious triumph over enormous odds are exactly what's digging our early graves, and hobbling us for years before the death that sadly many of us see as our only sweet relief. Just consider one element of this unskillful cultural heritage: excess. We do everything to excess. We eat giant burgers, drink giant beers, smoke giant cigars, and watch a giant amount of TV (on our giant TVs) over our giant bellies, all in service of our starving senses.

T. Colin Campbell, the Cornell University biochemist responsible for the single largest study of human nutrition ever conducted, devoted thirty-five years to studying thousands of people and interpreting thousands of other studies in what the *New York Times* called the "Grand Prix of epidemiology." He proved that in addition to diabetes and coronary artery disease, even leukemia and breast, colon, lung, stomach, liver, and childhood brain cancers are all directly related to what he calls the West's "nutritional extravagance."[2]

Let's talk extravagance for a moment. Someone I know just returned from a state fair where they were serving huge portions of deep-fried . . . wait for it . . . *Kool-Aid!* We pride ourselves on this kind of excessive ingenuity. Is it any wonder the Centers for Disease Control and Prevention in Atlanta predicts that *one in three* children born in the United States in 2000 will develop diabetes in their lifetime? For certain parts of the population most at risk, that number is one in two.[3] Is it any wonder we've forgotten what true, whole food tastes and feels like? Or what it feels like to get joy and satisfaction without 100 grams of carbs, 30 grams of fat, and that ineffable "purple" flavor?

Eating should be joyous. In fact, we're hardwired to enjoy it. If we didn't enjoy it, we'd probably avoid it and certainly therefore die. We should eat, but at the least begin to pay more attention to what we eat, rather than eating "mindlessly"[4] from the trough of deep-fried treats. We should stay conscious of the various ways food scientists and manufacturers—as well as those vendors at state fairs—pack in the drugs (literally) that short-circuit the pleasure centers of our brain to give us quick, cheap highs and help us forget the misery of our physical, spiritual, psychic, and familial lives for a fleeting moment. Believe me,

I'm sympathetic. I know it isn't easy. If you give a man cocaine for ten years, then pull him off it one day and expect him to get "high on life," well, you've got another thing coming. It's no different with food.

Ideally, we could attack this kind of cultural challenge head-on. That fits into my ideal future. Sure, deep-fried Kool-Aid, Twinkies, Pop-Tarts, and apple pie sound yummy to most of us, at least in the short term. But is it worth the kind of serial amputations diabetics refer to as "salami surgery"? Is it worth the worst pain you can imagine, radiating from your chest to your limbs, as you fall to the floor in front of your grandchildren from your third and final heart attack? I'm sorry to go to these extremes, but they're real, and edifying. As a physician, I'm honored to have been present at the deaths of many, many people. And in all that time, I've never once heard a dying person say, "You know, I wish I'd had more deep-fried cookie dough." What do dying people regret? Your intuition will tell you that it's not about satisfying taste buds. This whole book is about guiding you to a life in which you'll never experience that kind of regret on your eventual, far-off deathbed.

Meantime, it's imperative that we think about the easy and obvious things we can do today to prevent potentially horrific consequences tomorrow. We can drink enough water; lose some weight; eat whole, natural foods; get enough sleep; and eschew our tendency to revert to psychoactive substances or prescription drugs as quick fixes. That's a very, very good start. You can start all that today for no cost and very little trouble, and the results will likely be enormous. Many physicians would argue that you could do those things alone—you could stop reading this book now if you implement and stick to that prescription alone—but I don't agree. I believe you would certainly experience better physical health than your average citizen. But is that enough? Would it be meaningful? Could you even do it—sustain it, I mean—without a lot of support, not to mention the motivation and discipline that's often hard to muster? If you could, you probably would have already, it makes so much sense. I know it seems easier said than done, but I want you to trust me that you can start taking positive steps right away. Keep reading!

Ultimately, your health success depends on all the other factors of your life beyond your Pop-Tart intake, almost universally ignored in such prescriptions. It's clear we need to move well beyond this simplistic paradigm if we're to achieve a wonderful, long-term, nearly impenetrable sense of well-being. What's the point in keeping hydrated if you hate your wife? Why bother putting down the deep-fried ice cream if you can't stand your *life*?

Will conventional medicine come along with us for this ride into a more sensible and inclusive health paradigm? I hope so. We shouldn't give up on our doctors in this pursuit. On the contrary, we should hold fast to the expectation that our physicians should do more to guide us, teach us, and help heal us. Medicine in the West is a customer-service business, and the customer is king. If we start to ask the right questions, our doctors will eventually oblige and get with the program. But, in truth, we need to do a hell of a lot more to help ourselves, not the least of which involves embracing the broader slow medicine perspective on health and well-being, which I've been promoting. This doesn't have to come down to an either/or mentality, though. There's value in both the traditional, conventional way of practicing medicine and the holistic way. This is the "integrated" approach that makes the most sense, and carries with it the greatest hope for remarkable, life-changing, world-changing health.

9. Are All Your Senses Acute?

Remember, nobody's going to just hand you such extraordinary health. It's not up to your doctor. Because no two people are exactly alike, we must each discover our own path to health. Just as a violinist must tune his instrument to be in harmony with the rest of the orchestra, finding health is about discovering the right resonance or timbre within your own body and life. Once you're in the "flow," I promise you will know it. You'll *know* when you're healthy—all your senses will sing it out loud.

Identifying and developing your own innate strengths and skills is a good first step in finding the course that's right for you. Your own five senses and your sixth sense—your intuition—are already giving you messages from your body. You just need to learn to listen to them (not ignore their screaming) and properly translate the message to understand what they're telling you. Identifying and learning how to maximize these tools will be easier for some than for others, but the good news is that we all possess them.

GETTING IN TOUCH WITH OUR SENSES

Nearly all of us get to use our five basic senses every day. We taste our cereal, steak, and coffee. We touch our sheets and our spouses and our car seats. We smell our kids' diapers, the spring breeze, and fresh-cut grass. We see the mountain range behind the cityscape, the eyes of our dogs, the chiaroscuro in a Rembrandt painting. We hear a great drumbeat, the buzzing of a hornet, a car peeling out down the block. But how *consciously* do we use the tools of our senses? And to what end? Many people I meet—both patients and friends—take their senses almost entirely for granted, and use them for little more than day-to-day survival. It's not surprising that my patients who begin to *lose* their sight or their hearing suddenly recognize how much they value the simple things they once took for granted—how terrified they become at the prospect of no longer being able to hear or to see. They begin to speak of the emotional bliss they experience when they hear their grandkids laugh. They come to tears when they describe seeing the sunset.

So first and foremost, it's worth spending some effort on getting in touch with your senses, so to speak. Just a few minutes every day at first. Pay attention to the things you take in with your senses. Really *look* at the people on your commute to work, as the poet Ezra Pound did one day at the Métro station at La Concorde, Paris:

> *The apparition of these faces in the crowd;*
> *Petals on a wet, black bough.*[5]

That's amazing. One of the most powerful poems ever written in English, full of image, movement, elegance, transience, and profundity in just fourteen words, not one of them a verb!

Every day offers such poetic opportunities for all of us. For just a few minutes today, really listen to the wind outside, the brook trickling, the birds as they discuss their day. Hear kids giggling on the playground, distant, rolling thunder, or the battle cries in Wagner's "Ride of the Valkyries." Imagine for a moment the isolation, the loneliness that would ensue if this sense were suddenly snatched from you—then open up your ears again in remembrance that you are in possession of a sense that can immediately sweep your heart into a tumult of emotion with only a whisper. That's a miracle if ever there were one, and it's a sin to take miracles for granted, isn't it?

Attending, even temporarily, to our senses proves to us that regardless of any maladies we might suffer, we have incredible health right now—the ability to use all those powerful, miraculous faculties for experiencing the world around us. It reminds us that we're alive, and we're part of a big and interesting universe worth being a part of. You've heard the old wisdom: Open your eyes. Stop and smell the roses. Eat, drink, and be merry! Do it.

What does this have to do with extraordinary health? Well, on the simplest level, this practice promotes appreciation, which is paramount to good health. It helps us cultivate an "attitude of gratitude," as wise men and women—and SpongeBob, in one of his most popular children's songs—have suggested. When we appreciate what we see, hear, smell, taste, and touch, we are for that moment not focused on whatever other misery we might be enduring. We're actually *experiencing* health.

Think about how you would quiet a baby having a crying fit: jiggle some keys or walk over to show her some Christmas tree ornaments. We can entertain the agonized infant within us in the same way. It's not a *distraction*. It's a *focus* on what matters. On life. That's what I mean by a healthy relation to the universe.

10. Do You Take Time to Experience Sensual Pleasures in Healthy Ways?

My earlier diatribe against deep-fried state fair snacks notwithstanding, I'm not remotely an ascetic. I believe that good health includes experiencing the full range of sensual pleasures that God or evolution or chance has laid out before us. This is sometimes hard to achieve, especially if you want to achieve it with a measure of moderation, balance, or temperance.

On the one hand, we're assaulted daily with messages about satisfying our sensual impulses. From television and other media, we face an onslaught of images that provide a cacophonous feast for every sense. Images of juicy burgers and moist, plump cookies are meant to stimulate us. An eyeful of perfect supermodel-looking people in provocative poses and situations is meant to arouse other senses. The nonstop, pulsing clatter of media is meant to keep our senses stirred and shaken, forever off-beam. But at the same time, our still-puritanical culture encourages us to feel guilty when we experience—or even think about—satisfying such pleasures of the senses. We're taught at an early age to keep our hands out of the cookie jar, to keep our various pleasure-seeking behaviors in check. We're not supposed to put our hands down our pants. We can't stare. We can't eavesdrop on adult conversations. We're not allowed to say out loud when something stinks. We're trained to delay gratification and work toward "meaningful" feelings of satisfaction. That's fine. I get it. We have to live with others and learn to restrain certain impulses. And I think it's a good exercise to train ourselves to avoid substituting the kind of pleasure we might get from, say, illicit drugs or overeating, for real fulfillment that comes from something like inner peace or self-esteem.

I think we can make a good argument that many of us are in fact trapped on the physical plane, easily seduced by those things—like food, alcohol, and drugs—that bring us immediate gratification, despite their long-term negative effects. Our overconsumption and obsession with commercial and material goods in particular has bred a collective mindlessness, resulting in an avoidance of real meaning, real happiness, and real health. You know this. You can buy a sleek, fast motorboat and drink the best tequila. You can live in palatial home with a view of the Rockies unmatched by any Ansel Adams photograph. And you can still be miserable. A complete focus on the pleasures of the senses, absent meaning, can blind us to the wisdom that fosters an appreciation of the big picture, moving us into an even greater state of imbalance.

While contentment is the sine qua non—the indispensible essence—of peace of mind, we live in a culture that promotes its opposite. Advertisements make us feel incomplete, encouraging the endless pursuit of material wealth and sensual pleasure. We seek superficial gratification with little regard for its future consequences for the world or ourselves. We *attach* ourselves to things and people to avoid personal discomfort. We have conditioned ourselves to believe that satisfying all our wants, cravings, and desires will bring us happiness. The message is that we can have it all. Damn it, we deserve it all! Of course, the opposite is true. Our attachments and cravings, particularly to material wealth and temporary gratification, are actually obstacles to real contentment and real health. In fact, the mindless, mechanical pursuit of these things does nothing to address our underlying anxiety and simply perpetuates our fear and longing for something "real."

But I'm not talking about that kind of unbalanced excess here! I'm talking about an equal and opposite, unskillful and unhealthy problem. I'm talking about the danger that comes from inhabiting the other side of this continuum, where we get so caught up in our practical pursuits that we forget we have the capacity to even experience simple joy, fun, and pleasure from living through our senses: the fresh smell of rain or the majesty of watching a lioness romp with her cubs.

Get it out of your head that sensual pleasure is just for bacchanalian hedonists peeling grapes in their togas while slaves fan them with palm fronds. The simultaneous coolness and sting of a radish; the way the light plays on choppy bay water; the soft belly of a beagle; the thrill of a lover's touch—these delights belong to everyone. Life is greatly lessened if we avoid them. We certainly can't expect to experience extraordinary health without *sensing* the world around us in all its glory.

11. Do You Listen to Your Intuition?

THE ELUSIVE SIXTH SENSE

All cultures have a concept of a sixth sense, which we might loosely define as our *intuition*. Like our other five senses, many of us lose touch with this sense early on. This pattern typically starts with the reinforcement we receive from parents and teachers who unconsciously (or consciously) pick away at our confidence, slowly eroding our ability to think independently. When we're young, adults often dismiss our feelings and visions as fabrications or fantasies. They belittle us or ridicule our pride when our predictions prove true.

As we grow, more naysayers—usually because they are themselves insecure or afraid—keep labeling our dreams unrealistic, making us distrust what we feel inside is our truth. Collectively, these experiences lead us to distrust our deep inner sense of what's right for us. Eventually, many of us lose faith in our capacity for self-reflection and self-healing. When our confidence diminishes as a result, it's challenging to remain secure in our judgment and instincts, and this situation will affect our ability to make informed decisions about our physical, emotional, and spiritual health.

So we begin to turn outside ourselves—to peers, parents, bosses, the media, and "the system"—to solve our important personal questions and to lay out paths for our future. Our lives are conditioned— and in some extremes, controlled—by the dominant culture, the conventional wisdom, that makes us feel terribly insecure without "their" approval. You know: "They" say you're not supposed to get too much sun. "They" say you should spend three months' salary on an engagement ring. "They" say work is supposed to be a drag. "They" say you're not supposed to love this person or that one.

While there is some real wisdom out there, and while we can all benefit from a little guidance, we're bombarded by "experts" with definite, but not always transparent, agendas. We have become totally dependent on these others for advice. Perhaps this is why self-help books are so popular and appealing. It would be okay if we were able to consider such counsel in reasonable perspective, if we were able to keep the "self" part of self-help at the forefront. But over time we've continued to lose even more confidence in our own judgment and sensitivity.

This might seem strange coming from a health book author who definitely does want to offer advice. But I want you to be clear up front that what I'm offering is a method for you to truly *help yourself.* If you're seeking someone to take over the process of your achieving health and happiness, you've come to the wrong doctor.

But I understand the temptation. The world instructs us to follow conventional rules and norms of our society, so we do so, to fit in. But on some level, most of us *know* that society is out of balance with nature or even our own most precious values. But we learn early on that we mustn't upset those at the top or the masses around us. Over time, we get used to these prescriptions and proscriptions, and find it easier to just go with the flow rather than creating waves. Notice, though, that when every once in a while a true self-possessed maverick comes along, we call such a rebel a hero. Those people change the world.

And the rest of us? Basically, we've become lazy. (If you object to the word "lazy," perhaps you can substitute "asleep" or "unconscious.") In any case, we sit back and wait to be told what to do instead of figuring things out for ourselves or using our own creativity to solve problems. We allow other, often less skillful people to influence our minds and behavior. That's the definition of bad advice. Part of the reason we're so susceptible to such bad advice lies in our vain quest for easy answers, to locate the "Idiot's" or "Dummy's" guide to all our problems. This quest stems from our acquired fear that we can't trust or rely on our instincts.

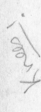

While confidence in ourselves is in short supply, often our confidence in others is equally low. We might expect other people to bring us to our goal, but we often find that they're flying as blind as we are. Even those in whom we place great trust, or to whom we turn for guidance—our leaders—ultimately let us down, sometimes with devastating consequences for our psyches. We all know what happens in Washington, D.C.; how often the "hope" of the election season turns into the "nope" of petty politics. In fact, this has become a sad joke, a reflection of a society that has become truly numb to hypocrisy.

In his renowned essay "Self-Reliance," Ralph Waldo Emerson spoke eloquently of the need to rely on our present thoughts and impressions rather than those of other people. He urges us to trust ourselves, for "God will not have his work made manifest by cowards."[6] Emerson stresses originality, believing in a person's own genius and ability to discover resonance from within. The human hunt for self-reliance, he says, is really a search for harmony in the universe, which can be achieved only by each person seeking his or her own unique means of self-fulfillment (here substitute "health" and "wholeness").

So how do you find your own, unique and authentic self? Try turning off the faucet of others' advice for a bit. Trust your instincts. Find quiet moments to sit and listen to what your inner voice tells you that you must do to feel better, to be wiser, to live more meaningfully. The more you connect with your deeper self, the more confidence you will find in your own perceptions and intuitions. Wake up your senses! Get outside. Adjust your diet so it's more in harmony with what you know is good and right and healthful. Spend more time with your family the way you know you should. Mend relationships with lost relatives and friends the way your inner voice is calling you to. Start a good book you've been intending to read. Pursue your callings. Ignore the words of leaders who are misleading you. The more you do to empower yourself, the less power you will give away or lose in the process.

Let me reiterate that: stop giving energy and power to those whom you suspect (your intuition tells you) are not reliable or trustworthy. Whenever possible, limit your exposure to the negative messages that produce fear, anxiety, and shame. Learn to be more discriminating about the voices to which you listen, about who and what is feeding your brain. Get in touch with your *self* and listen to what it's been

telling you all along. This is an imperative step on the staircase to
extraordinary health.

> ## 12. Are You Relaxed and in a Calm
> ## State of Mind When You Eat?

WHAT'S ON YOUR MIND WHEN YOU EAT?

Let's get practical. All of this takes a lot of thought. It wouldn't make
much sense to care so much about what you feed your brain if you
ignored what you put in your belly. But you should understand by
now that the brain and belly are both part of a single integrated system. Perhaps the most essential element for the individual in pursuit of
health is to understand what *nourishes* and *sustains* us, both physically
and metaphysically. For that reason, it's critical that we consider how
to make the best use of the sources that feed us on every level. We
need to explore the concept of "conscious eating."

For the most part, food pundits and "experts"—although well
intentioned—have overcomplicated the process of eating, leading to
neurotic tendencies and frankly crazy behavior around food. I think
it's essential that we relax about food, because worrying about food is
causing as many problems as eating the wrong kind of food. I would
like to suggest that we *enjoy* our food as well as the company dining
with us. I'd like to prescribe that we maintain a sense of gratitude and
appreciation for what we eat, for all that goes into that food we consume. And I'd like to recommend that we don't overthink every food
choice we make. People have gotten so caught up with the science of
nutrition that they've forgotten the art of eating.

This is not to say that we shouldn't think at all about we what eat.
I subscribe to the notion of "conscious eating," about which many

nutritionists, psychologists, and health authors have pontificated lately. However, in my mind, conscious eating is about more than just the specific foods you choose to eat, important as those choices are in terms of long-term health.

No, the kind of consciousness I'm talking about goes deeper—it's about the choices you make about yourself in general and your health in particular. It's about the way you consider and treat your *self* as an entity in the universe. Yes, it's true from a health perspective that we are what we eat, but the underpinning and the real meaning of conscious eating is actually something more: assuming you're not simply eating Twinkies all day long, what's on your mind when you eat is as important as what's on your plate.

There's so much worthy advice out there about how to eat well to avoid disease and improve health that I hardly need to review it. In fact, I'm willing to bet that not a single reader out there remains unaware of the basic parameters of a healthy diet. You already know most of the things you need to do for better health. We all know, and we *know* that we know. Yet look around your average shopping mall, flea market, or sporting event. Do your neighbors and relatives and coworkers look like they're practicing what they know very well? Are they listening to their intuition about skillful eating? I don't think so. Why is that? There's clearly some paramount consideration beyond common sense that compels many of us to ignore the obvious repercussions of our bad health choices. Perhaps we just feel as if we deserve to treat ourselves. And the treats that really seem to satisfy give us a short-term high (from excess sugar, fat, caffeine, alcohol, nicotine, and so on) that helps us ignore the long-term low that follows if we abuse them.

Suffice to say, we're not really hungry for a pint of double chocolate fudge ice cream, but hungry instead for some feeling of wholeness and happiness and joy that we can't seem to find anywhere else—so

Häagen-Dazs will have do. In other words, we're hungry for health. We're just scooping from the wrong bin.

THE THREE KINDS OF HUNGER

We can review the practical "diet" part of this program pretty quickly. It will dramatically improve your overall health if you eat regular, moderately sized, and balanced meals, heavy on fresh and seasonal high-fiber fresh fruits, vegetables, and whole (unprocessed) grains, and limit excess animal products and processed food that contains unnecessary fat, salt, sugar, and chemicals. That's it.

The only problem with this perfectly sane and sensible prescription is that practically no one is complying the way they should be. As a result, the rates of diseases caused by poor diet choices are skyrocketing in this country. If you've tried typical weight-loss diets such as Atkins and Weight Watchers, and found they don't work, you're not alone. Most people I see have at one time or another been on a diet. Very few are successful over the long term. What I want you to appreciate is that good health and nutrition are not as simple as prescribing to you an ideal set of foods that will make you healthy. Generally speaking, you're not eating poorly because you're physically hungry. In fact, there are three kinds of hunger: physical, emotional, and spiritual. If you think about your needs that way, it might open your eyes to a new perspective on eating. See, the problem is that we often confuse these three types of hunger. Rather than considering which hunger we're feeling at a given time—much less *why* we're feeling it—and attempting to understand the distinction between these hungers, we just "feel hungry." So we eat. Usually some kind of unhealthy "comfort" food, specifically designed to change our brain chemistry in the same way that cocaine and heroin do.

If we're *emotionally* or *spiritually* hungry, having not been able to "feed" ourselves effectively in those areas, then it seems to us that our only source of fulfillment for the *sensation* of hunger will be from food. But guess what? It doesn't work! If a car needs gas, no amount of oil will make it go, and vice versa. So we get more emotionally or spiritually hungry, while at the same time, we've stimulated more physical hunger by releasing those chemicals in the brain that then compel us to eat more junk. It's a vicious cycle.

Instead, imagine if you could address your emotional and spiritual hunger in a more skillful manner. Working this way, there would be no reason for a diet at all: you would simply not need to eat so much, and what you desire would be more in line with what is really best for you as well. It's a win-win.

So don't worry—this is not a book that will chide you for having a burger, fries, and shake *once in a while.* Yes, I'll remind you about some basic choices you can make that will likely improve the way you feel right away. But you'll also discover a whole new world of extraordinary health once you think beyond the conventional—when you think about how satisfying your work is; whether you have a purpose or mission in life; the extent to which you feel connected to a life force like God; and how in tune you are with the rhythms of nature. Inquiring into these things and making incremental improvements in these areas, even as we care for our bodies, can have dramatic and lifelong positive effects.

When we start to work on these oft-neglected areas, we achieve a sense of well-being and a legitimate quality of health that can generally withstand some less than ideal choices about what we do with (and to) our bodies. If you're deeply in love and happy with your mate; if you serve your community and feel useful in the world; if you wake with gratitude every day—then your health can probably handle a few extra pounds, a beer or two, some chocolate, or the occasional bowl of Cherry Garcia (but maybe not the whole pint in one sitting, tempting as it is). I've found that in many cases, patients who work the 77 Skillful Questions tend to find it a lot easier to make better choices about their physical bodies. A patient recently came to me at SunRaven with pretty serious work and family stress. He found that as he began using techniques for keeping calm and centered, he felt compelled to rebuild his diet, too. He'd been consuming a lot of sugar and junk food, which of course was stress induced. And as he began to incorporate more whole and natural foods, some of his other physical symptoms—headaches and intestinal issues—began to abate. I see this all the time.

In other words, when your relationships with your past, your spouse, your boss, and the world around you are fulfilling, you tend not to seek fulfillment at the bottom of a Häagen-Dazs pint. When we do a careful inventory of why we're hungry, we begin perhaps to *respect* ourselves more. We find greater worth in taking care of ourselves. We're excited about our lives, and we're no longer so "starved" for fulfillment, seeking to satisfy that starvation in sweet, fatty, salty places.

EATING WITH YOUR BRAIN ON

Along the lines of conscious eating, I have a few other food-related suggestions for you in your pursuit of better health. It's in this context that the value of locally grown, whole, sustainable, and seasonal food can best be appreciated. It's not just about the nutrients, but the fact that thinking this way takes into account the entire food chain and all the consciousness that goes into every aspect of raising, delivering, and preparing the food that we ultimately consume. If and when all the links in that chain are working in a healthy and sustainable way, we folks at the top of the food chain are more likely to achieve the health we seek.

When you grow some of your own food, you are forced to be conscious of every aspect of the food chain. But whether or not you have the means to grow your own food, you can develop the knowledge and resources you need to get nourishment from where it's most beneficial. When you couple this with a mind-set that learns to be at peace at the time when you actually sit down to eat, you're on your way to healthy eating.

Let's think further about the concept of the food chain. It's one thing to eat foods we all know are healthy, but another entirely to focus on where those healthy foods come from, how they're made, and, most important, what conditions maximize their nutritional value. A person who makes skillful food decisions has the potential to receive more "nutrition" (in the broadest sense of that word) and to simultaneously live more skillfully by positively affecting all life on our planet. Eating with awareness sets you up for a more enjoyable and wholesome dining experience. To paraphrase an old Hindu mealtime prayer:

The creative energy in the food is divine,
The nourishing energy in the body is divine,
The transformation of food into pure consciousness is divine.
If you know this, then any impurities in the food you eat
Will never become part of you.

At one time or another, we have all engaged in unskillful eating habits. To make the point, here is a graphic example of an unskillful food practice: veal production.

Typically, handlers separate young male cattle from their mothers immediately after birth (females are reserved for breeding and milking). The male calf is then chained in a two-foot-wide wooden crate and kept in darkness most of the time. The calf can't turn, stretch, groom itself, or even lie down comfortably. Significantly, it's not

allowed any interaction with other calves. Because the goal is to produce the pale, flabby meat that we consumers prefer, ranchers deliberately ensure the calf becomes anemic by feeding it an iron-deficient
formula free of the roughage that's part of a cow's natural diet. Because
the hungry calf would desperately eat any hay bedding, it has to lie
on a bare, slatted wooden floor, covered with its own waste. It would
seem miraculous that any animal could survive in these conditions.
And in fact, only a diet of antibiotics and other powerful drugs keeps
the calf alive for its brief, unpleasant life span. Even so, many calves
die, and others are so ill or feeble at sixteen weeks that handlers have
to drag them along the bloody ground with hooks to their slaughter.

Sorry if I spoiled your appetite. Many people find the practice of
veal crating so odious that some countries have banned it outright.
While a small proportion of ranchers raise veal calves with "ameni-
ties" like hay bedding and the opportunity to eat and interact with
other animals, this "humane" treatment is more the exception than
the rule.

I'm not saying that you should give up veal. That's a personal
choice that I respect either way. What I am suggesting is that you
develop an awareness of the circumstances under which your food—
all our food—is produced. In this way, you start to cultivate a *consciousness* about what you're putting on your plate and in your body. In
my view, this gets us much closer to a state of health than mere adher-
ence to some specific and restrictive diet. Having said that, developing
a consciousness about the circumstances of food production will tend
to redirect a person's food choices away from unhealthy options and
toward more wholesome and sustainable ones. If more people visited
hot dog–making facilities, a lot fewer people would eat hot dogs.

I'm not trying to bash meat here, either. My suggestion is that
you honor the entire food chain. In the case of vegetables, for example, think about all the work and the people involved—from the seed

supplier to the farmer and the farmworkers. Reflect on all the effort required to harvest the plants and to pack, store, and ship them to their final destination. Imagine the hours spent each day stocking produce aisles. Along the way, scores of fellow humans—often overworked and underpaid, but that's another book—have expended a monumental amount of energy and effort just so you can buy an avocado, or a bag of "baby" carrots (typically just regular carrots machine-cut down to miniature size). It's important to mention that anywhere along this journey, not only the environment but also the conditions of the workers can variously "pollute" your food. And the process itself can be harmful to both the humans involved and to the environment.

Have you ever caught a fish and cooked it over a campfire? Or grown your own tomatoes and sliced them up for a salad? Anyone who has knows well that such food simply *looks* and *tastes* better, and makes you *feel* better. It's very likely that without any processing or pollution, such fresh and whole food is, in fact, healthier. You can experience this for yourself by gardening if that's possible. If you live in a city or otherwise don't have property, consider a simple herb garden or a window box for a few choice veggies. Or look into a local community garden. Community gardening projects open acres of land, often in the middle of urban areas, to the entire neighborhood, allowing volunteer participants to learn to cultivate organic, biodynamic, and sustainable crops, and to gain a mindful awareness of nature that promotes personal and collective growth and overall community and ecological health. Plus, it's a lot of fun, and you get to meet cool people who share a community-minded ethic.

In my experience, these projects are particularly allied with health and slow medicine because they encourage participants to celebrate seasonal cycles, such as the equinoxes, the solstices, and the full and new moons, helping to align us with the forces of nature. Here again, the value of the produce that results is important, but perhaps secondary to the benefits of working in the natural world to sustain our families and the human family. If you don't have a local community garden, why not start one?

But you don't have to go to such extremes to start a healthier, more conscious eating program. You can start by supporting local farmers over mass supermarket chains, or simply by trying to understand more about where your food comes from. The idea is to come into alignment with everyone and everything around you that contributes to the food you ultimately choose to eat.

Whatever you eat, you should *honor* your food, and see how this honor affects your overall experience of eating and your health in general. Consider how they do it on Sardinia, off the coast of Italy, for example. There, the typical diet consists of homegrown fruits and vegetables, dairy products from grass-fed sheep and cows, home-baked flatbreads, fresh fish, and wine produced in small vineyards from indigenous grapes (writing this is making me hungry!). Sardinian families, generations of whom often live under one roof, typically eat together, and the stereotypical celebratory atmosphere of the Italian table is no fiction. Sardinians typically involve themselves in every step of the food process, from planting and growing to harvesting and cooking. Interestingly, more men live past the age of one hundred on this Italian island than anywhere else in the world.

Some experts suggest that a healthy, low-stress, agrarian lifestyle is the main reason why Sardinian centenarians have outlived most of their compatriots in urban and suburban Italy. Others suspect that genetics underlies the unusual male longevity, which appears to run in families, but of course, if genetics is the cause, it might just be the result of thousands of years of this relatively stress-free, rural lifestyle centered on the whole-food diet. Whatever the true explanation, this overall conscious, simple, skillful approach to food that many traditional agrarian societies take is worth emulating if you want to "live long and prosper." So, *mangia!* I know this is probably not what you expect a doctor to tell you in a chapter that includes a prescription for healthy eating. Instead of succumbing to restrictive rules and regulations, focus, starting today, on food *consciousness*. Ask the following kinds of questions before meals:

- *Where* did this food come from?
- *Who* was responsible for it?
- *How* did they make it?
- *What's* in it?
- Can I still recognize what it *used* to be?
- *How* did it get to my kitchen or this restaurant?
- *Why* do I want to eat it?
- In *what way* am I hungry?
- How am I *feeling* right now as I'm about to eat?
- How will I *feel* soon and later if I eat it?
- What are the likely *consequences* to my health if I eat it?
- What are my other food *choices* right now?

Finally, when it does come time to eat, try to foster a peaceful and loving energy to surround your meal. Think about joyous and grateful times when you've shopped for, prepared, cooked, served, and eaten your meal with people you love. Not every meal and snack will automatically have that kind of energy, I know, but meditating for a minute each time you eat—such as certain religions intend when people hold hands to say grace—will help you to make better choices, eat better, digest better, feel better, and live better. Then, as you take your first bite, turn off the voice of judgment inside your head and enjoy what you have chosen for that moment.

13. Are the Environments You Live in Clean, Pure, and Conducive to Health and Peace?

. . . .

CLEANING UP YOUR ACT

This one's pretty simple. Use your senses and your intuition to assess the relative healthfulness of your immediate surroundings. You know now you need to turn off the spigot of bad advice around you to reconnect with positive, healthy intuition. You know you have to stop the flow of unhealthy food to open yourself up to better choices. Well, so, too, should you stop the tide of negative physical influences and strive to surround yourself with as pure, clean, and natural an environment as possible. What circulates around and in your body affects what you get out of that machine.

When you think of your environment, what comes to mind? Be honest: Are your kitchen and bathroom less than pristine? Is your bedroom full of dust? Is your workplace akin to one of those veal-fattening pens I just described? Are you, like many modern workers, suffering in a cluttered cubicle under fluorescent lights, permeated by the stench of copier toner?

You wouldn't go out of your way to drink filthy water, would you? So why would you deliberately breathe bad air? Or subject yourself to other "toxins" in your surroundings? Truth is, every drop you drink and every breath you take that contains pollutants and toxic chemicals will ultimately foul up the machinery of your body and tax your systems as they attempt to clear those poisons. So cleaning up the environments where you spend the most time— your home and your office—is a prime opportunity to improve your overall health.

This is not just a good idea—it can literally save your life. Research shows that a quarter of all disease in the world is caused by environmental factors, and environment plays some contributing role in a full 80 percent of all diseases, according to the World Health Organization.[7] Unhealthy environments kill a staggering thirteen million people a year,[8] often through diseases of the respiratory, digestive, hepatic (liver), and blood systems. Nearly all of these diseases are preventable by cleaning up environments—primarily our air, water, and household toxins. In the most extreme cases, in sub-Saharan Africa, for example, where diarrhea and malaria are two of the most common killers, poor environmental conditions take nearly 100 percent of the blame. But these factors affect us in the West as well. A large body of recent evidence points to significant indoor environmental contributors to asthma, for example.[9] Exposure to toxins in the home and workplace can cause or contribute to lupus; Parkinson's disease; reproductive problems; any number of cancers, such as mesothelioma and breast cancer; and a range of other serious diseases and conditions, including, possibly, autism.[10]

Just use your intuition and your common sense. Don't you feel better when you get fresh air? When your sheets, your toilet, your countertops are clean? When you eat more wholesome, unprocessed, natural foods? Doesn't the sun feel healthier than artificial light?

Here are a few simple suggestions for purifying your environment in pursuit of better health:

- Eat wholesome, natural, unprocessed foods.
- Consider eating organic where possible.
- Grow some of your own fruits, vegetables, and herbs without pesticides.
- Drink plenty of fresh water, filtered if you're concerned about your local source.
- Clean your house regularly of dust, dander, pests, and other allergens.

- Consider getting a HEPA air filter.
- Limit your intake of poisons such as nicotine, alcohol, and illicit drugs.
- Limit your exposure to toxins such as chemicals in the household (room deodorizers, for example) and at work.
- Reduce your use of toxic chemicals on your body, from fragrances to strong chemical antiperspirants.
- Pay particular attention to the cleanliness of your bedroom and your desk/office, where you spend most of your time.
- If your pets sleep in your bedroom, keep them and their bedding constantly clean.
- Don't forget to avoid noise and light pollution whenever you can; these can have serious negative effects.
- If you don't have control over your work environment, take frequent breaks, especially getting fresh air whenever you can.
- Get moving! Physical activity can help rid your body of environmental toxins.

Just as important as the physical issues relating to pollution is the benefit that can be derived from mindfully adjusting your environment to be more in alignment with the overall principles of slow medicine. In this regard, intentionally adding beauty to your environment, or arranging the furniture of the rooms in which you spend a lot of time so that it's most conducive to work, rest, peace, harmony, or whatever else you are doing there, will contribute substantially to your state of ease, balance, flow, and productivity, all of which are essential components of the health you're after. The Chinese call this feng shui, and for four thousand years, they've put it to good use.

You've heard the phrase, "Clear desk, clear mind"? Well, this is quite true. In the same way, a healthy environment makes for a genuinely healthy person. Further, when you clean up your personal space, you're actually serving others at the same time. After all, we share the planet with each other, not to mention every other living thing.

PRACTICAL PRESCRIPTION 2: FINDING TREASURE

At this point, I suggest that you try an interesting experiment on your path to integrative health. Try thinking of every day of your life as a kind of treasure hunt. There are moments each day to find various treasures, literal and figurative—even during periods of suffering. You can use your senses to unlock these treasures. As you navigate the path of your life, physical conditions might persist and pose challenges. However, you should always keep in mind that the physical realm is just one component of health. Yes, your trick knee can hurt like hell, but it doesn't diminish the brilliance of your husband's smile. Your nose might stay clogged today, but that doesn't eclipse a gorgeous sunrise.

You might even be facing the gravest of health challenges, waiting in hospice for imminent death itself, and still find wonder, joy, and appreciation in the things big and small beyond yourself—a tiny spider laying eggs in the corner of the ceiling, the sound of bullfrogs in a distant stream, a Beethoven symphony, the memory of your first kiss. I understand it's often difficult to transcend physical and emotional problems—but it's very much worth trying. It's "healthy" in the best definition of the word.

If you open your heart and mind, you'll find that very often, the journey of life presents critical opportunities to bring even more meaning and beauty into your life. You just have to look out the windows once in a while as you ride through life to see the meaning and beauty radiating from those you love and who love you; the meaning and beauty you can sense in the wonders of the earth; the meaning and beauty of your dreams, imagination, and hopes for yourself and others. The hope that springs from your intuitive sense of where you could go if there were no obstacles.

If this sounds corny or silly to you, I urge you—I beg you—to give it a try. How about you look for treasure for ten minutes a day? How about for three minutes while you brush your teeth or wait for a red light? Spend this time daily considering and truly appreciating such meaning and beauty, and I guarantee you will feel better, happier, more whole, more balanced, more in tune with the world—in short, healthier.

Are you asking, "What *&^%# treasure? My shin splints are killing me! My bunions are the worst!" Well, how about treasuring the time you have alone on the cool tiles of your bathroom as the sun streams in and you notice in the mirror that your eyes remind you of your beloved father? How about treasuring the nonstop, stupid, loyal love of your dog when she sees you're awake and ready to take her for a walk? How about treasuring the miracle that your faculties are intact; that you can dream and picture wonderful things for your grandkids and even yourself? How about treasuring the mystery of the future? Whatever happens, it's going to be a surprise.

There's treasure, too, in embracing who you are on your unique journey. Finding health requires a personal transformation that's not accomplished by blindly following others toward short-term goals, but by going after the ultimate state of peace and tranquillity—the real treasure. And you can't find peace and tranquillity if you're running away from yourself. Can you find a kernel of something to treasure about yourself right now? It's one of the saddest heartbreaks that many of us believe we cannot. It takes practice; it doesn't come naturally. It feels selfish. It feels prideful. Bull! You're cool. You've done some interesting things. You've overcome a lot. You've touched people. You've left a mark. You've learned stuff. You have a heart and a mind and a soul and a body, all imperfect, but all yours, and all wonderful and awesome, in the true definitions of those words. Please, please, for just those three minutes while you wait on the bank line, allow yourself to feel this instead of gritting your teeth in frustration. If it works, maybe expand this practice to your evening ablutions. Then maybe every time you find yourself on hold with customer service. Then whenever you're about to go to bed, and so on. Look for the moments—they are there.

If you're still uncomfortable finding treasure in yourself, think about others. Think about your friends. Think about soldiers. Think about firefighters. Think about children. Think about horses. Think about God if that's consistent with your beliefs. Think about the formation of the sun and the planets, quarks and quasars, black holes and red dwarfs and dinosaurs and all the sponges bobbing in their brown shorts below the sea. Think about your favorite stories from childhood, your favorite jokes, your favorite cookies that your grandma used to make.

Note that it's difficult to find treasure when you're constantly putting out fires. Too often we're focused on the thousands of tasks at hand throughout our overly busy days. We move so fast that we lose sight of the beauty that surrounds us. We're so busy looking for our kid's socks that we forget the profound, almost painful love we feel for them. We're so intent on finding our umbrella that we forget how lovely the rain feels on our faces. Remember when you were a kid and the most fun thing you could think of was to jump in a puddle? Exactly when did we change our minds about that? And what good did it really do us to grow out of it?

Again, for most of us, this practice will not come easily and will not work perfectly right away. We're so conditioned to find fault, to focus on problems, to concentrate on pain, that some of us go our entire adult lives without finding any treasure. How do you hedge against this worst of tragedies? Well, this might sound morbid, but imagine that today's the day you will die. (We ought to have learned

from recent events that it very well might be—we just never know.)
I think the vast majority of us, given twenty-four hours or even one
hour, would not simply curl up and wait for the grim reaper's sickle.
We would deliberately and passionately seek the treasures in our
lives. Our senses would come alive, and we would not take them for
granted. We would savor the touch of those we love. We would make
love if we could. We would feel profound love for those who've supported us, and we might even find forgiveness for those who've "trespassed." We would relish the breeze on our face, or the brush of our
cat's tail against our leg. We would feel the pulse in our arteries and
the breath in our lungs, and find them astounding. I can assure you
that we wouldn't worry about getting our Hush Puppies muddy—we
would jump headlong into any puddle.

Funny thing is, we don't typically find such treasure, in part because
we don't believe today should be "a good day to die." Today feels like
just any other day, and, frankly, today kind of sucks. But does it really?
Open up your senses and you'll find that it's amazing. It's awesome. It's
a miracle. It's plain common sense.

QUESTIONS FOR FURTHER REFLECTION

14. Are You Grateful for the Blessings in Your Life?

15. Do You Feel Physically Attractive?

These two questions are worth some additional thought. Actually,
they require practice. Can you learn to draw your attention to the
positive and to accept all that is? Can you see light and beauty even in
the shadows? This is worth the effort, I can assure you.

3

CONNECTING WITH NATURE: UNDERSTANDING HOW IT ALL WORKS TOGETHER

. . . I have felt
A presence that disturbs me with the joy
Of elevated thoughts; a sense sublime
Of something far more deeply interfused,
Whose dwelling place is the light of setting suns,
And the round ocean and the living air,
And the blue sky, and in the mind of man:
A motion and spirit that impels
All thinking things, all objects of all thought,
And rolls through all things . . .

—William Wordsworth[1]

I'D LIKE TO CONTINUE THIS DISCUSSION—your consultation—by asking you to tune into the greatest teacher we have: nature. Here, the questions are going to focus on the world around us, and how we interact with those things we see and otherwise experience every day but rarely connect to our own processes. In our highly mechanized and structured age, we've become dangerously disconnected from this world, and from the cycles of life of which we should feel a "natural" part if we expect to experience extraordinary health. I want to remind you what your intuition already knows about the idea of these cycles and their relationship to health. I want to show you how to get yourself more in alignment with the natural world and the way things are *supposed* to work. Once we really look into the fundamental rhythms and cycles of human life, such as sleeping and waking; working and resting; conceiving and dying—life and death—we start to appreciate a deeper resonance with nature that's foundational to a new and true definition of extraordinary health.

HEALTHY BY NATURE

I'm not proposing that we all get naked and dance in the mud—although, apart from the potential for trichinosis, that's arguably not at all bad for your health. I'm suggesting that you think about the natural environment and its observable cycles and rhythms, but also its largely hidden yet powerful flow of energy. Aligning with these forces is an instant remedy for what chronically ails us.

My slow medicine prescription includes that remedy, which most doctors simply ignore. It represents good medical science synthesized with many wise traditions, among them Taoist, Vedic, Native American, and ancient Greek, all of which share the core understanding that there are not one, but two fundamental aspects to the human condition: the physical body, which consists of our bones, organs, glands, blood, and so on, and, *as significantly,* an energy source that actually animates the physical body and the rest of the living and nonliving things in the universe. I understand that it can be challenging to marry the traditional and nontraditional approaches to health and healing, but I have learned that this is required for wholly integrated health.

Think about it this way: You're floating down a river and you have only half a paddle. Or maybe you have a whole paddle, but you're trying to paddle upstream. Either way, you're wasting valuable energy, and the extra effort produces heat and inflammation in your body *and* prevents you from achieving the health you desire—that ideal state, where purpose and harmony coexist. While recent advances in technology and scientific knowledge have helped us gain a measure of "dominance" over nature and the physical body, to the point where we can actually alter our appearance, gender, and even our genetic makeup, it's precisely the promise that we can change nature that has led us to neglect some primary facts about our human condition and our potential. In other words, these scientific achievements have come at a price. Today, many, if not most, of us have lost sight of our very *nature,* and as such, are suffering more pain and disillusionment and purposelessness.

I have spent decades trying to better understand our connection to the whole of nature as I work on becoming the best healer I can be. Here's one of the things I learned in my quest to become a skill-ful gardener: if we carefully observe how nature works, we realize that many things that at first appear "broken" or "imperfect" are not. And for those things that do need repair, we come to understand that the "fixes" don't necessarily come from an outside source. In fact, the capacity for healing resides in all of us. Take forest fires, such as the ones that are devastating the Colorado mountains as I write this chapter. From the point of view of a tourist hoping to see a verdant, lush forest, such fires seem destructive. But both ancient wisdom and modern ecology teach us that regular cleansing fires are essential to the long-term health of any forest. While the destruction of homes is tragic, terrible infernos are, in fact, completely necessary for a place like Yellowstone to become as beautiful as it is in the first place. Only after the fires there in the 1980s did experts understand that it took some 450 degrees Fahrenheit for the seeds of the great lodgepole pines, the emblem of the Yellowstone landscape, to germinate. Our ideas about "perfect" and "imperfect" are often affected by whether or not we take a look at things from a higher vantage point than we're used to, from a more holistic perspective. That includes trying to see things over longer courses of time—the antithesis of the instant-gratification/quick-fix mentality we've been trained in. If we see the fire as emergent and calamitous, and we respond by putting it out, we put the long-term, *natural* future of the forest in peril. Our egos and our technology have gotten in the way of a natural process.

We do this with our bodies as well. Let's look at fevers, for example. When our child has a fever, our first reaction is to make it go away at whatever cost (some doctors call this "fever phobia"). We make three critical mistakes in this kind of thinking:

1. First, we don't usually question the *source* of the fever. A fever is just a symptom of a systemic body problem. What's going on in the child's life that might need attending to? What have they come into contact with? Could they have some inflammation, such as an abscess? An infectious disease like the flu? A metabolic disorder like diabetes? An immunological disorder like juvenile rheumatoid arthritis? The vast majority of fevers are relatively benign, so I'm not suggesting parents should "catastrophize"[2] them and assume the worst. But before thinking about making the fever go away, it's a good idea to wonder why it's there in the first place, how it might be the body's right and natural response to a problem. If all we do is try to get rid of the fever, we might miss its value.

2. Second, we act against nature. When it comes to one of the most common causes of fever, infection, the body's autonomic nervous system, seated in a clever gland called the hypothalamus, has developed an elegant healing mechanism: it raises the body's temperature to kill many kinds of pathogens and to allow infection–fighting white blood cells to move around more freely in search of the invading organisms. With the exception of very high fevers (105 degrees and up), which can cause serious damage to the body and therefore require immediate treatment, fevers, like many forest fires, should run their own course. Using unnatural aids to reduce fever (aspirin, acetaminophen, and ibuprofen) typically *prolongs* illness rather than shortening it, even while ignoring the cause.

3. The third problem we run into is that we train the child in the quick-fix mentality that has gotten us in our present medical mess, and we reinforce it in ourselves. We "put out the fire" and alleviate some discomfort (really, we just mask it), but neglect the long–term health of the human "forest." We need to cultivate patience and an appreciation for the growth opportunities inherent in certain states of discomfort.

Yes, a fever can be unpleasant. But lots of water, ice pops, and a fan can ease the unpleasantness while the child's body naturally heals itself. During that process, perhaps the child can benefit from the brief sabbatical from his or her busy and stressful life. Gone are the days of chicken soup and a hug as the underpinning of treatment—even though those treatments really do serve the child's health. Sadly, we live in a world where our pharmacist's prescription has become more important than our mother's love. How's that working out for us?

Don't get me wrong—our interest in minimizing acute pain and suffering is understandable and valid, as is our initial desire to put out the fire in the forest. But a skillful study of nature reveals that the solutions we need will not always come from applying technology, but are often best guided by inner wisdom; in particular, the pursuit of learning, growth, and *meaning* we go through in investigating a challenge, even when we realize up front that a "cure" is not available. In this regard, there's often something good that can come from the "forest fire." In fact, the capacity for healing (the ability to find meaning that leads to "wholeness," a process akin to evolution, in any situation) resides in all of us.

Again, the slow medicine approach here is to develop the skills, asking and answering the right questions, to make the best use of all our tools and deploy them in ways appropriate to the circumstances. The typical Western mind-set, by contrast, tends to favor the physical cure, while placing the inner learning process on a second tier or discounting it entirely. I'm suggesting that we try to transcend those limited models. Ideally, we learn to use both. After all, in our very nature, we possess both sets of tools.

16. Do You Think of and Treat Your Body as a Series of Unrelated Parts or a Whole and Unified System?

THE BODY IN SYSTEMS THEORY

In my town, it's all about horseback riding, but when I go out for a walk, I often see the diehard cyclists tackling the Westchester hills. One day, I stopped to talk with a competitive cyclist whose teammates had left him on the side of the road because of some problem with his bike. This machine cost more than my car, but it was hobbled by a tiny problem—some cable somewhere had snapped. This got me thinking about the "health" of a machine, and how the whole system's function depends on the interrelation of its parts.

A bicycle is an organized system of constituent parts, such as a chain, handlebars, a frame, pedals, and all those cables going back and forth. Now let's dismantle it. Let's grease every piece, and polish them until they shine, then lay them out on the side of the road. We can argue that we no longer have a bicycle per se in front of us, but merely a collection of parts that has the *potential* to be a bicycle. You see, it's only when the bike is assembled properly—when all the parts work together, playing their "part" in the whole operation—that it functions as a bike. In fact, if we look only at the individual parts, we often fail to view the potential system they create once we put them together. If we saw any heap of parts on the side of a road or a shop floor, we might miss their intended purpose altogether.

Now, you know where I'm going with this. The same principle is true of the human body, of course. But it's also true of the greater system of life within which the body is situated. Whether or not you believe in God, evolution, "intelligent design," or random, lucky happenstance, it's hard not to concede that we live in a world—and we live in bodies—engineered to work as complex systems constructed of organized and interrelated parts. Understanding the relationships between the components both within the body and between the body and the surrounding systems is critical to truly mastering ourselves, to truly making us function optimally—to our *health*.

Thinking otherwise about our health strikes me as the height of reductionist and unscientific thinking. The functional quality of your whole system is the most important measure of your health. In other words, if your pedals are working but your tires are flat, you're not the best bike you could be.

It turns out there's some very sophisticated science out there that studies this principle. It's called systems theory, and it tells us that in any system, the interaction of component parts is as important as the parts themselves. You don't have to tell that to the cyclist who had to ditch his bike, nor any physician worth his salt.

However, since the age of seventeenth-century philosopher René Descartes, modern medicine has clung tightly to the limited and limiting belief that "matter" is separate from "spirit." This is like saying the bike and its *purpose* are separate. Indeed, four hundred years later, this way of approaching the body has led to great advancements in medicine. However, when Descartes separated matter from spirit, the body became seen as a mere machine. This is a powerful metaphor, because it suggests that the body can be objectively known through science, and therefore technically fixed by a skilled mechanic. A physician fixing a body, in this context, is akin to a bicycle mechanic repairing a broken chain. While well-intentioned, this Cartesian view about health seems to assume that eventually advances in technology will be able to fix anything and everything that might get broken in the body, to save us from any disease or faulty engineering we might encounter. Well, despite that promise, this view of life and health has great limitations. Something seems to have been lost. For one thing, we've lost sight of the body's delicate interrelatedness with the natural world in which we exist, with the greater living system in which we are embedded.

This way of thinking, which reduces something to its smallest parts, is known as reductionism for a reason. This myopic view of health leads to the expectation, among patients in particular, that every affliction has a definitive cause, awaiting discovery by medical research or diagnosis and cure by a physician. These ideas form the subconscious cultural context out of which much thinking about health arises, at least in the West. But can you really optimize a bicycle chain without understanding how the gears and the wheels and the pedals work with it? And what happens when the chain and the pedals and the cables all work—but the bike just doesn't function as well as it could? What do you "fix" then?

If you think about it, an organized system *can* function perfectly well (though perhaps not optimally) if *certain* parts are on the blink. The cyclist could have gone on with his ride if a few spokes of his wheel had bent, or even if he'd lost the seat or part of one pedal. Yes, a system functions best when all its parts are working well, but when the whole system is functioning well, it can often stand a few rusty, busted, or missing parts. The same is true of the body. Just look at all those champion athletes with fewer than the *optimal* four limbs. Would you describe a para-athlete as "unhealthy"? This is an important distinction: you *can* experience Olympic health with a missing leg, but not a missing heart. Conventional medicine often disregards this distinction, and so do we as patients. Embracing slow medicine and working the 77 Skillful Questions will help you understand both how to eventually integrate all the aspects of great health and how to triage the few critical aspects you must get a handle on as soon as possible, lest you wind up in the ditch.

Real health will come only when you recognize that symptoms often reflect *systemic* challenges, which might or might not even be directly related to the part where they *seem* to reside. Imagine going to your bike mechanic saying there's a problem with your wheels not turning. Sure, there might be something stuck in a spoke. But, even more likely, there might be a problem with the gears or the chain or the pedals (or the rider!). In the slow medicine paradigm, all the parts are connected in a whole system and play a role in its function. Moreover, what's on the mind of the rider? What are you doing and where are going with your machine?

17. Are You Conscious of the Causes of Your Physical Conditions and Aware They Might Lie Outside the Body?

BODY, MIND, AND SPIRIT SCIENCE

Now, let's take this one step further. In the same way all the parts of the human body are interconnected and interdependent, so, too, is the physical system of the body connected with its other systems, such as the emotional and spiritual. There's a lot of narrow-minded thinking out there about health care. To some in the über-conservative camp, it might seem preposterous to have patients consider factors such as their relationships with their children and parents when diagnosing and treating a health problem like migraines. Some would say that's not good science. Influenced by my traditional medical school training, I, too, might have fallen victim to this insular and reductionist way of thinking. But, faced with the assertion that going beyond the physical is too out there to be considered real science, I applied rationality, as I assume you will, too. Ask yourself: Do I care about what uninformed, limited thinkers believe about holistic philosophy and methodology—or do I care about achieving health? How do I feel after applying these principles? Isn't that the basis on which you grade your health and your health care, from F to A? Of course it is. And what grade are we getting right now? You remember.

Irrespective of limited thinking, when you report that you *feel* better, then you *are* better. You experience a better quality of life. You can do the things you want to do without restriction. You feel more hope and more freedom. You feel more of a sense of purpose. You certainly feel more in *control* of your health. When, along the way, your symptoms abate or disappear completely, then that sure seems like health. I don't care whether critics call that science or magic or voodoo.

Don't get me wrong. In no way do I believe in the kind of medical shams and scams that promise complete cures for serious diseases from such and such a supplement, magnetic patch, crystal, or "balancing" bracelet. Nor can I brook the kind of manipulation that puts desperate, vulnerable people into a state of denial or fantasy that ignores basic realities of their physical bodies. Your intuition should tell you that this faith-healing tactic is usually more about filling the donation basket than fulfilling parishioners' or patients' health.

We're not talking about that kind of stuff here. Here, we're talking about the fact that there is more to our health conditions than mere physical symptoms. I'm going to say that a lot in this book, in several different ways. Repetition leads to automation. The mind-body connection is self-evident, in addition to being proven, scientifically, time and again.

So the next consideration for achieving extraordinary health is to ask yourself whether you already know intuitively what might be causing or contributing to your symptoms. When it comes to most acute health problems, there's often an identifiable physical cause. A gunshot wound to the thigh will hurt in the thigh, and a plan that removes the bullet, treats the wound, and fights infection will often suffice to heal the physical condition. But it's pretty rare to have a *chronic* health problem with such a singular and obvious physical cause. More often than not, we have to go beyond the physical to find all the contributing factors and develop an optimal treatment.

It's amazing how often and how well my patients are able to use their intuition and their other senses to diagnose the causes of their health problems, and to recognize that many sources of symptoms are situated outside the physical body (with no magic bullet to remove from the thigh to ease the pain). You've done this yourself, I'm sure. Sometimes it's as simple as recognizing that stress lies behind tension headaches or exhaustion leads to colds and flu. But just as often, it's more complicated and unique to each individual. Starting a new job, going through a divorce, dealing with financial problems, excessive travel, even moving houses can all contribute substantively to knocking the body's natural systems out of balance. The resultant health problems, though they arise out of *systemic* stresses originating on the nonphysical planes, might manifest themselves in any number of specific parts of the body, causing pain, inflammation, weakening, or other symptoms, some of which can debilitate you. It's worth noting that the parts of the body where the symptoms settle can indeed be relevant in diagnosis and treatment, and many cultures' traditional medical philosophies have studied these connections in detail.

But no amount of treatment targeted at your frozen shoulder will properly heal you if you don't unfreeze those other aspects of your life situation that might lie behind that specific body part's immobility. Are you feeling stuck at work? Are you trying unsuccessfully to move away from a relationship? Are your feelings about a given painful situation at a standstill? (Note that the roots of the words "motion" and "emotion" are identical.)

18. Do You Take Walks, Garden, or Have Other Regular Contact with Nature?

NATURAL ENERGY

As you can see, the basic premise of my idea of health is rooted in the idea of *interdependence*. You've seen how our body parts fit together to form a unified whole. And you've gotten a glimpse of how our physical body and our mental/emotional state are related. Now, let's go beyond. I know as both a doctor and an avid gardener that good health requires us to experience a powerful recognition that we humans exist within the entirety of life here on our planet. Very often, when we feel "unhealthy," it's because we're unbalanced, unconnected with (or resistant to) the natural order—an understandable but regrettable by-product of our modern age. Ironically, it's our age that made the kinds of advances that prove we're literally *made of starstuff.* When we remember that—when we live in alignment with the rhythms and cycles of the natural world—we discover balance, fulfillment, and growth, a wholeness that we can define as extraordinary health.

Therefore, the next phase in healing is to try to bring yourself more into alignment with natural rhythms, cycles, and processes. This is easier than it might seem at first blush. The first step is as easy as an *actual step:* I suggest you step outside.

Is your intuitive answer to this question about feeling empowered by nature something like "Are you kidding me? I spend fourteen hours a day in the office"? Then you already know intuitively that there's something out of whack. You know that despite scores of years and billions of dollars spent on ergonomic workplace designs, we humans were simply not built for fluorescent lights, desk chairs, computer monitors, and fourteen-hour days of reconciling balance sheets.

19. Do You Feel Energized or Empowered by Nature?

TAKE TWO SQUIRRELS AND CALL ME IN THE MORNING?

My prescription for nature is simple. Go out and enjoy it on a regular basis. Most of us are so unskillful in this area that we probably need to retrain ourselves to enjoy nature as we did when we were children.

Why do so many of us fail to find contentment in the simple act of walking in a sunny park, looking at birds, squirrels, and trees? In fact, instead of absorbing the wonder of the natural world, many of us are likely to covet the things we encounter while we wander through the park. We're shopping with our eyes. We see a new bicycle, a sleek pair of sneakers, a jogger's iPod. We direct our focus and attention toward *objects,* which will never provide true contentment and certainly have nothing to do with extraordinary or even ordinary health. This is part of the cultural pathos in the West, which began a few thousand years ago with the simplest of technologies that eventually led to the domestication of animals, master manipulation of crops, and super-processing of foods. These developments were wonderful in some ways, allowing us all kinds of modern conveniences.

It's quite nice to not have to slaughter a bison yourself for dinner. But in many ways, these advancements have regressed our health. Earlier cultures could not store grain for months on end and needed to hunt and gather every day, which helped foster a cycle in their daily life that was very much in alignment with nature. Our modern society has moved far away from this rhythm for the sake of convenience and freedom. The irony is that we're actually more constrained now—and certainly less healthy in some critical ways. In fact, most modern chronic diseases are diseases of overdevelopment, overprocessing, overabundance, overindulgence. In short, we're not dying of starvation anymore. It's just the opposite. Look around for empirical proof.

I'm not suggesting that you abandon all modern conveniences and luxuries, even though living a simpler existence might move you closer to nature's rhythms. I'm just talking about reconnecting to those things that are more inherently fulfilling—such as loved ones and the bounty of nature—rather than fleeting material possessions like your Lexus and your Jet Ski. This can move you into a more balanced and healthy state. By reprioritizing and letting go of the accumulation mind-set, which keeps many of us stuck in habitual patterns of unskillful behavior, we start moving to the rhythm of our world, which we must do to rest comfortably in our authentic nature. Think of the connection between the words "heal" and "whole."

A great place to begin this healing is in the great outdoors. A park. A lake. The woods. Even your own backyard. Like many children who were raised in suburban America, I have fond memories of climbing trees, playing in leaf piles, wading through shallow brooks, and spending leisurely afternoons fishing with my father and grandfather. But as *New York Times* journalist and child advocate Richard Louv writes, an entire generation of children is at risk now of growing up without such memories. Today's child, says Louv, is more adroit at identifying SpongeBob than any native species of plant or animal, and overwhelmingly prefers computers and video games to a sandbox or tree in the backyard. Louv calls the physical, emotional, and cognitive disconnect from the natural world "nature-deficit disorder."[3] This disconnect from nature, he asserts, is evident in the recent increases in childhood obesity, attention deficit disorder, and depression. On top of this, children are learning from parents, teachers, and the media to literally *fear* nature: *The sun causes cancer. If you lie on the grass you might get bitten by a tick. Jellyfish sting!* All this fear and avoidance exacerbates the dearth of unstructured, healthy, natural activity in the life of today's child. You don't have to be a doctor to know it's not healthy. My prescription: Go out and play!

Both children and adults who either feel or really are disconnected from a vital source such as nature, family, or the divine are ripe for various sorts of overindulgence, in a vain effort to fill that void. It could be food. Drugs. Sex. Material goods—doing "retail therapy." Such excess inevitably leads to a never-ending cycle of fear and emptiness, of agonizing longing. Anyone caught in this paradigm will eventually spiral out of control. Falling out of balance leads to poor health and *dis*-ease.

On the other hand, those who are connected to a vital source and create a vital existence through contact with each other, with nature, with the planet and its resources, are likely to lead a more fulfilling, stable, and healthy existence.

Sounds potentially complicated, but it's as simple as turning off the TV, getting up from the desk, getting out of the easy chair, getting out of the car—and getting outside into nature! There are many critical benefits of a regular engagement with nature. You don't have to tackle K2 or swim the English Channel to get these benefits. You just have to take walks, or garden (my preferred method), or build snowmen on a regular basis. Here are just three of the huge benefits of getting out in nature:

1. Increasing your physical activity can and will have benefits on your overall health: it reduces inflammation, lowers blood pressure and blood sugar, increases endorphins, and helps you lose weight, just to name a few.

2. Regular, limited exposure to the sun is good for you: it increases your energy for the day and will even help you fall asleep more easily. Physiologically, it will convert vitamin D to its active form, helping your bones stay strong and your immune system fight cancer and other diseases.

3. Outdoor activities, whether alone or in groups, calm the nerves and ease stress: they create a perfect opportunity for peaceful reflection and meditation.

20. Do You Engage in Regular Physical Activity, and Are You as Physically Strong as You'd Like to Be, with Good Endurance and Aerobic Capacity?

. . . .

MOVING RIGHT ALONG

There's no escaping it: Good health won't fall on you while you're sitting on your sofa. You have to move—literally—toward a healthy life. The idea that physical activity, even the moderate kind, is a key to achieving good health is so well understood that it hardly warrants an explanation. Except for one thing: you're probably not doing it. At the least, you're not doing enough of it. It's a strange paradox. Your intuition—not to mention the collective wisdom of thousands of years of study and observation—makes it clear that if all you do is get moving, you're likely to improve your health, perhaps vastly. Yet all the "modern" conveniences of our world keep your butt more and more firmly planted in your car, your desk chair, or your couch. You're looking for advice on improving how you feel? Browsing Web sites and buying books? When all the while you know you're not burning enough calories, getting your joints limber, and pushing sugar out of your blood and into your cells where it belongs, simply by moving around a bit, preferably outside? What's stopping you?

There are a few things. For one, the myth that you have to go whole hog to get any results. Sure, a strong and consistent regimen of hard work over the long haul will likely cause massive improvements in your health. But chances are you're not up to that. Perhaps you are somewhat—or even very—out of shape. So does that mean it's too late? Your exercise should consist of vending-machine-button pushing and chip dipping? Every fiber of you knows that's not going to cut it. So how about something in between Rocky's training to fight Apollo

Creed and the average American's quest for Couch Potato Champ? Even Ralph Kramden bowled and danced a little now and then!

What I'm suggesting is small bouts of physical movement, on a regular basis. Although it's wise to maintain somewhat physically challenging goals, you can work up to those, so you don't injure yourself early on or decide to give up because the "pain" is more obvious than the "gain." Here are some ideas. Perhaps some will look familiar. If so, I'd suggest you find one that pushes you to the next level.

- Park the car in the farthest spot from the store and *walk*.
- Take the stairs and not the elevator.
- Walk the dog instead of just letting him out. Or offer to walk an elderly neighbor's dog.
- Play catch or go sledding with your kids or grandkids.
- Go bowling, dancing, swimming, or mall walking with friends.
- Mow your lawn.
- Garden, rake leaves, or plant trees.
- Go for a hike—there are plenty of flat trails to get you started. Then, start walking up some hills.
- Pick up the pace when you do housework.
- Take a bike trip to a favorite picnic spot (pack some seasonal fruit from a local farmer's market).
- Clean up an overgrown lot in your neighborhood.
- Take an evening stroll to look at people's holiday decorations.
- Volunteer to paint a playground wall.

Of course, I strongly favor the kind of physical activity you can do outdoors, whenever possible. But the key here is movement first, for a sustained period. If you need a number, start with twenty minutes.

But if you can't do that right away, do what you can, then see whether you can incrementally build up to twenty minutes. The second key is regularity. While fly-fishing once a year is better than never, it's not enough to get appreciable results (and short bursts of intense activity after long periods of sloth can lead to injuries). Can you do twice a month, though? How about every weekend? The third key is to mix it up. You'll get bored, even by your favorite physical activity, if you do only one thing, over and over. So how about walking the dog at least once a day, playing golf on Sundays, and hiking with friends the first Saturday of every month? Then you can fill in other activities as they come up.

An interesting facet of physical activity is that it's self-motivating. Getting the juices flowing—as long as you don't push it and exhaust yourself—makes you more likely to want to go again. It could be those famous endorphins—molecules released by the brain when you exert your muscles. It could be the sun. It could be the self-confidence you gain by regular movement. It could be your chronic conditions abating, or some combination of all these things. In any case, when you move, you move toward health. Just about every major and minor health challenge will improve with regular movement. Most notably, movement will decrease inflammation, the condition at the root of the Big 8 health challenges.

You don't necessarily need to train for something specific. You can just enjoy the movement. But many experts suggest that specific short-, medium-, and long-term goals can help motivate you. So maybe you want to take a bunch of short hikes in preparation for a longer weekend of hiking at a local mountain you've never been to. Maybe you want to take increasingly longer walks with your dog to get ready for a dog-walking charity event in a few months.

When you're ready, you can step it up. If you're moving long enough and actively enough to sweat a few times a week, you're going to see faster and more noticeable results. All this conservative talk about taking it easy doesn't mean you can't aim big. My seventy-five-year-old father still keeps himself in shape—among other reasons, so we can take exotic fishing trips, such as the one we just took to the far reaches of Chile.

SUNNY DAY

How much time have you spent in the sun recently? I bet it's not a whole lot. In our endless pursuit of obeying what "they" say is good for us and bad for us, we've fallen out of balance with the natural order. You know, the much-maligned sun seems to have served us pretty well for a few million years of human existence. But all of a sudden, in the past thirty years, we've come to think of our local star as Mortal Enemy Number One. Many a respected medical professional has warned us sternly about the dangers of that yellow monster in the sky.

Yes, there is such a thing as skin cancer—and it can be deadly. This kind of cancer can occur as a result of *excessive and repeated* exposure to direct sunlight. In my medical opinion, however, I think it's wiser to get outdoors more, without worrying too much about the risk of skin cancer. I know this might sound counterintuitive or contradictory to prevailing medical wisdom—you might even think I'm crazy. But there is no such thing as life on Earth without the sun. You *need* the sun: it's the only way to convert vitamin D to an active form the body can use. Humans require vitamin D for a healthy skeletal structure and immune system, among other things. So I'm not suggesting you strip and scald yourself all summer, year after year, with no protection, as they did during the golden age of sun worship. But neither do you have to retreat into lotion-slathered, shady fear. Soaking up a few rays of sun after lunch, the way cold-blooded animals do, is a good and healthful activity, in accordance with natural law. It's a good idea to get some sun on your skin and to expose your eyes to a little sun during the early part of the day (take off your UV blockers): this will help you release more melatonin at night and fall asleep without supplements or sleep aids.

21. Do You Fall Asleep Easily and Soundly, and Do You Wake Up Feeling Rested?

HITTING THE PILLOW FOR HEALTH

Over the past several centuries, our society has drifted away from a way of living that's supported by nature's rhythms. We eat when we should be digesting, we speed up when we should be slowing down, and we "spend" when we should be "saving." And perhaps the most noticeable and potentially egregious flouting of natural cycles is our ignorance of the *circadian* rhythm. In short, we are too often awake when we should be sleeping. And when we do sleep, it's irregularly, restlessly, not enough, or too much.

Adults in the United States average just 6.7 hours of sleep a night, and 43 percent of adults use a sleep aid several times per week, according to the National Sleep Foundation.[4] Up to sixty million Americans cope with sleep disorders such as sleep apnea or chronic loss of sleep.[5] Perhaps only one-third of American adults get enough sleep every night.[6] I bet it's even fewer. A new report by the Centers for Disease Control and Prevention shows that more than forty million workers in the United States get less than the minimum six hours of sleep per night that doctors recommend.[7] This causes thousands of on-the-job mishaps per year, not to mention about 20 percent of all car accidents.[8]

As you can imagine, it's very big business between your sheets.

The sleep market is worth $23.7 billion, and it's growing nearly 9 percent a year. Companies that market major anti-insomnia drugs such as Ambien, Lunesta, and Rozerem spend $619 million on advertising and produce $2.7 billion in sales every year.[9] They're gently assuring you with luna moths and dream-beavers that there's a solution to this common ailment: pop a pill and fluff your pillow.

Sure, we need better sleep, but not with drugs. How do we do it? The first step is to fall more into line with the daily cycle of nature. The circadian rhythms are tied to the day/night cycle of Earth, sun, and moon that determines the eating and sleeping patterns of most animals (including, up until recently, us). Brain-wave activity, hormone production, bone growth, cell regeneration, overall healing—and even weight loss, to some degree—are all tied to this daily rhythm, and totally reliant on us regularly shutting down shop, preferably at night. Our bodies have their own circadian rhythms, too, which work on the same schedule, more or less, as the day/night rhythms of nature (in other words, a twenty-four-hour clock) in order to regulate other body systems. It seems we're hardwired this way, and for a reason.

The circadian system relies on regular, rhythmic periods of light and dark to keep everything in sync. Contrasting light/dark is the most important cue for your internal rhythm, essential for the adequate production of critical hormones like melatonin, cortisol, testosterone, and even growth hormones, all of which work to keep your complex body systems regulated and in balance. What happens when it's not in balance? Think about jet lag. If you travel far out of your time zone, your body will respond with confusion. You might experience fatigue, loss of appetite, or disturbance in bowel movements. Basically, you're out of rhythm, off cycle, lagging.

But as a culture, we're experiencing a *mass* jet lag, occasioned by short-circuiting nature. In the old days, you had to go to bed when the sun went down, because you couldn't see enough to work at night. You got up with the sun to get back to the farm or the hunt or the family. Sleeping and waking with the sun and the roosters might not be totally practical in the modern world for anyone but farmers (though the resident peacocks at my home, SunRaven, daily try to persuade me otherwise)—but the closer you can get to achieving this rhythm, the better for your health.

Nowadays, however, our society has completely discounted the normal rhythms of day and night that the brain needs in order to properly trigger the coordinated torrent of hormonal and neurochemical reactions that are necessary to the processes of building tissues and muscle and in repairing organs and DNA, and in the regulation of weight and mood chemicals. We do this with all-night TV, Internet, and video games; shift working and workaholism; caffeine, alcohol, and other stimulants; and regular, excessive sleeping in when we should be awake and enjoying the sun, nature, and our daytime lives.

But perhaps the biggest challenge to circadian rhythms is the advent of constant artificial light throughout the evening and night. This disrupts the body's natural circadian rhythms, often with dire consequences in the long term. It's a terrible but typical paradox that perhaps the most important invention in modern human history is also one of the most destructive to our health. In particular, artificial light, especially at night, wreaks havoc with melatonin, the hormone that helps make sure you have a good night's sleep. Melatonin is produced in your pineal gland, a tiny, highly evolved, pinecone-shaped gland in the center of your brain. When your eyes sense the bright light of a sunny day outside, they transmit a "lights are on" message to the brain, which in turn shuts off the formation of melatonin. As it begins to get darker outside, the eyes send this update to the brain, which instructs the pineal gland to kick up the melatonin production again. Here's the most interesting part: the pineal gland uses as its building block for melatonin a neurotransmitter called serotonin—the molecule that's produced in the body by exposure to natural light during the day. This is why you tend to sleep better at night after you've been outside and exposed to a lot of sunlight, such as after a long day at the beach. Your serotonin levels are soaring, and as the day turns into darkness, your melatonin levels will soar, too. It's good night, Irene. To help this process, you can eat a diet rich in tryptophan, as that's the basic building block of serotonin. That's why you feel sleepy after a heavy meal of tryptophan-laden Thanksgiving turkey.

A sidebar on serotonin: Do you know what the most common class of prescribed drugs is? If you said "SSRIs," you're right. What does SSRI stand for? Selective serotonin reuptake inhibitor. Depression and serotonin are related. The serotonin your body makes today expires every night, so you need to expose yourself to outdoor light every day.[10]

No surprise then, people who don't get enough sleep tend to be depressed more often,[11, 12] which can have devastating consequences on overall health and can lead to other conditions of equal danger. Good sleep can even reduce chronic diseases:

> Good sleep also helps ease the diabetes process. Dr. (Karine) Spiegel of the University of Chicago found that healthy young men had 40 percent lower blood sugar uptake by their tissues (meaning their blood sugar was higher) when they got only four hours of sleep for six consecutive nights than when they had six nights of adequate rest (contrasted to the six nights before, during which they got enough rest). Further, insulin released from the pancreas was 30 percent lower after sleep deprivation than after nearly a week of adequate rest. And the ability of blood sugar to enter body cells without help from insulin dropped 30 percent, to a level usually seen in type 2 diabetes. In short, sleep deprivation left healthy young men with an

ability to handle blood sugar comparable to that of an elderly person
with a mild form of diabetes. One explanation is that loss of sleep
appears to raise stress hormone levels, which in turn may increase the
body's resistance to insulin, leading to more difficulty bringing blood
sugar into tissues.[13]

Studies have even shown an association between a disruption of
circadian rhythms and an increased risk of cancer. Studies conducted
by the Agency for Research on Cancer showed that healthy circadian
rhythms played a critical role in cell cycles, DNA damage response,
and tumor suppression.[14] Besides contributing to depression, diabetes,
and cancer, circadian rhythm disruption can also increase the risk
of obesity, cardiovascular disease, and other serious, chronic conditions.[15] So hit the pillows.

Try turning down the lights and going to bed early. Avoid caffeine and any activities that energize you in the evening. For example,
if you're easily roused, it might not be best to watch a scary movie,
the news, or any kind of high-energy TV late at night. Even a normally healthy practice like yoga might not be ideal too late in the
day if the asanas (postures) you're performing stimulate the adrenal
and pineal glands, both of which are related to light and the waking
state. Instead, consider more relaxing postures after sundown. Finally,
if you're still staring at the ceiling and counting far too many sheep,
make sure your bedroom is totally dark and keep your room cool.
The contrasting warmth under the blanket will actually make it more
conducive to the sleep you desire.

When I studied under Dr. Andrew Weil, he talked a lot about the
importance of good sleep for healing the body and lowering susceptibility to illness. Dr. Weil identified the overactive mind as one roadblock to
good sleep, and suggested a "relaxed breath" technique akin to meditation or self-hypnosis.[16] Find your own techniques for quieting the mind

and body at night. As you progress through the 77 Skillful Questions and begin to come to terms with your larger life issues, I believe you'll find it easier to fall asleep more quickly, stay asleep more soundly, and wake more refreshed. It's a huge foundation for extraordinary health.

PHASES OF NATURE

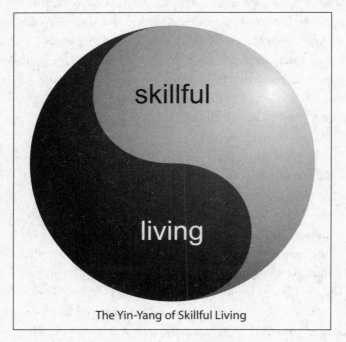

The Yin-Yang of Skillful Living

We understand and can easily accept that cycles exist everywhere in nature, including its history. At one time or another, our Earth has been boiling, frozen, stormy, volcanic, pacific, desiccated, moist, and everything in between. It's been teeming with life and utterly desolate. The ground where my home sits in Westchester County, New York, was once a vast ocean swarming with exotic fauna. People often lament global climate change and the other environmental catastrophes taking place on this planet. Those concerns are certainly serious, especially as the generations living today have actually been witness to some rapid and alarming changes. Yet, in the grand sweep of time (give or take 4.5 billion years), the planet has seen far greater catastrophes, and will see far worse in time to come.

I don't want to dismiss the potential problems associated with global climate change, particularly as they might be caused by our abuse of the planet. But to label these events as purely "bad" is to deny the essence of our existence. All these disasters and upheavals reflect normal cycles, which actually have brought us to this place and to this moment in time. Looking at it from an evolutionary perspective, if a meteor had not slammed into the Yucatan 65 million years ago, wiping out nearly 90 percent of all living species, then perhaps our proto-human ancestors wouldn't have found the wherewithal to emerge into the former stomping grounds of the dinosaurs. Perhaps you and I might never have existed.

If glaciers hadn't scraped across our continents and lava not bubbled up, had mega-quakes not rent the landscape, we wouldn't have had this amazingly beautiful and bounteous world we live in.

More recently, looking at the human toll, the epic tragedies of Hurricane Katrina, the Indonesian tsunami, and earthquakes in Haiti and Japan were truly awful. Huge numbers of people lost their lives, their families, their homes, their livelihoods, the very core of who they are. The emotional toll was quite significant to countless others. As a doctor, all my instincts to help kick into gear when stuff like this happens. The desire to ease pain tops my list. However, from the point of view of all nature and the history of life on this planet, it's worth asking—after we've tended to hurting humans—whether all these events are really objective "tragedies." Are they all necessarily negative, in the larger picture? We are so invested in survival that we view every extinction, flood, tornado, eruption, and hurricane as a calamity.

But nature itself is indifferent to the processes it sustains. The great wall of water that refills Africa's Zambezi River after the long dry season also floods crops, drowns unsuspecting animals, and destroys nearly everything in its path. Who among us would not watch in horror as a pack of hyenas snatched a newborn gazelle from its mother's watchful gaze? Are these hyenas killing for sport or pleasure? Or just to feed their own offspring? Nature's moral relativism is hard for Westerners, in particular, to comprehend. Because so many of the processes that sustain one life also take life away from another being or species, it's impossible to determine whether something in nature is purely good or purely bad. I recognize that many of us don't do well with this level of ambiguity. And I understand that if it had been my home destroyed by Superstorm Sandy, or my children, God forbid, killed, I would certainly see this as bad.

But I also see that the strict good/bad dualism of the Western mind-set puts us at a disadvantage. In fact, it distances us from nature. Our ubiquitous Judeo-Christian model polarizes us: good/evil, moral/immoral, heaven/hell, and so on. By contrast, the Taoist yin/yang diagram, the Vedic mandala, and the Greek Ouroboros (the snake that eats its own tail) acknowledge distinct entities, but each emphasizes interconnectedness, interdependence, and flow. The yin/yang symbol doesn't resemble one of those black-and-white cookies you get at an old-fashioned New York bakery, split perfectly down the middle. Instead, you see each side rounded, bulging into the other, and there's always a little piece of one side in the other.

Perhaps the great sages of these ancient traditions were saying that life's opposites are merely expressions of a deeper underlying unity; a cycle that connects and defines life in all its forms and processes. Instead of choosing black or white "sides," perhaps it's more skillful to investigate how ostensible opposites actually merge into one another, as in the forest fire scenario. This is the true definition of the word "reconciliation," which means to restore the circle or whole. Restoring the circle or cycle allows for the integration of opposites, "in blunting the sharpness and untangling the knot," as the ancient Chinese philosopher Lao Tzu writes.[17] Nature effortlessly moves toward this homeostasis, or balanced state. This is why nature is *the* archetypal model for Skillful Living.

You can see that we've abandoned our ancient appreciation for nature's cycles. We spend our energy craving and cultivating wealth, power, and privilege when we should be craving and cultivating enlightenment and peace. Making more money to buy even more things to acquire "contentment" is a cherished way of life in the West. Industries produce and sell goods and services for enjoyment without relation to need or the quality of life. More goods and services generate more demand for more things; advertisements fuel the demand for things we do not come close to needing. And the more things we feel we need, the more we need to work. This vicious, man-made cycle is at odds with natural rhythms both in our world and within ourselves. When we get caught in that trap, we take away from others, we deny our true purpose, we sacrifice real health and happiness—and we strip the planet of its resources, polluting our air and water, to boot. That's what's known as an unsustainable system. We must reconnect with the rhythms of nature for our bodies, minds, and spirits to work well within the natural order. I can absolutely guarantee you that without ever directly addressing your knee pain or your TMJ, if you work *this* treatment, you will feel better.

FERTILITY: HOW FAR OUT OF RHYTHM HAVE WE GOTTEN?

To exemplify how out of sync with nature we've become, let's look at fertility for a moment. How big a problem is infertility? According to the National Center for Health Statistics of the Centers for Disease Control and Prevention, about 12 percent of women between the ages of fifteen and forty-four (7.3 million) in the United States have difficulty getting pregnant or carrying a baby to term.[18] These numbers mark a profound increase from when I was born in 1960. Why has there been such an increase in the numbers of women—and men—requiring extraneous intervention to conceive a child? Have we rapidly evolved somehow? Not quite. But our bodies have certainly adapted to the new way we're living, largely contrary to natural cycles.

Infertility is one of the more common medical mysteries plaguing modern society. I've often wondered about the origins of this growing trend, considering that life, as we know it, would come to an end without conception. A closer examination reveals distinct patterns to the infertility we've been witnessing. For one, there's a lot more stress in our ambient environment. There's a lot of talk surrounding stress-related fertility suppression, which is based on the observation that many couples achieve pregnancy after adopting a child, stopping fertility treatments, or making significant lifestyle changes. There's a valuable clue! But many medical experts are likely to dismiss such incidences as anecdotal, and because they can't easily be quantified, they're generally not studied or looked at seriously by researchers. However, it's commonly accepted in environmental and population biology that fertility is suppressed during times of great stress such as famine, drought, or disease. Could you imagine a gazelle trying to conceive during a drought, or a zebra becoming pregnant while running for her life from a pack of hungry lions? As we are animals who are just as much a part of nature as zebras, it seems unlikely that our ability to reproduce would not be affected by corresponding environmental and psychological stress as well. What are the hungry lions in our lives?

Moreover, because more than one-third of all infertility cases are idiopathic (having no known obvious physical cause), it's possible that even many of the medically identifiable causes of infertility such as hormonal imbalance, pathology, and low sperm count are stress related or otherwise *psychogenic* (not originating in the body, but arising out of mental states).

The world is moving at a very fast pace—a fact reflected in the day-to-day lives of many people. We travel, dine out, work, and socialize outside of the home far more often than people of my parents' and grandparents' generations. Like the zebra, we always seem to be "running," not from lions but from the Lions Club, to golf with the boss, to the PTA meeting, to do all the errands necessary to keep up a modern existence on the grid. In other words, we devote a great deal of time to nondomestic activities. Interestingly, the word "domestic" comes from the Latin *domesticus,* which means "belonging to the house." Is there any bird that lays its eggs before it's built a nest? Would a polar bear give birth before she's dug a den? How many of us in today's hectic world feel really *settled* at the point when we wish to bring a baby into our "nest"?

JANE'S STORY: THE VALUE OF SETTLING DOWN

I have a patient, Jane, who, like many modern American women, was having troubling conceiving. At first glance, it seemed odd that she would have trouble at all. She was trying to get pregnant at the biologically appropriate and vital age of twenty-nine; she had a successful and fulfilling career as a high school basketball coach and physical education teacher; and she was in a loving, stable, and happy marriage to Owen, a businessman with a flourishing career in international finance. She appeared healthy on every level.

However, some clues to her problem came to light as we spoke further. For one, Jane's job, while fulfilling and enjoyable, required her to do a great deal of traveling, taking her away from home a lot more often than she and Owen would have preferred. Similarly, Owen's job also necessitated frequent trips, and he was often away for long stretches. On those rare occasions when they were together, Jane and Owen seldom spent any time at home. They ate out often, and always socialized with friends in restaurants and other people's houses, when they weren't taking care of their various chores and duties.

Moreover, the place they called home was not really a home at all, but a temporary residence where they'd essentially parked their stuff and themselves while waiting to settle down "later." See, neither Jane nor Owen was certain they would or even wanted to stay in their current house. What was the point of settling in when they both knew that at any time they might have to pack up and move to accommodate the requirements of Owen's career? As a result of this uncertainty, they didn't consider themselves part of any neighborhood or community. They didn't really get to know any of their neighbors and didn't feel that they could count on anyone nearby as friends.

Furthermore, even if she did conceive, Jane worried about how she would fit a child into her busy schedule of work and socializing and other obligations. In this respect, she was similar to many professional women I meet in my practice.

As Jane relayed her story, I was struck by how similar it was to that of our ancestors who might have worried about bringing a child into the world after a particularly arduous winter when food was in short supply. Although their lives were very different, their physiological responses were identical. If worry is the prevailing thought and energy coursing through a woman's body—if she feels both physiologically and psychologically unsettled—then it makes sense that some natural mechanism could hamper fertility. Starvation-induced stress was the prevailing factor thousands of years ago. Things are no different today; it is just a different kind of stress, and another form of starvation.

Despite these concerns, Jane and Owen really wanted to have a baby, so they decided to undergo many months of invasive, painful, and costly fertility treatments—a whole panoply of new stresses. Even the most up-to-date, cutting-edge techniques involve high doses of hormones and/or manipulations of the body. Hormonal hyper-stimulation of a woman's ovaries and procedures such as transvaginal egg retrieval carry significant risks. In vitro fertilization procedures increase the likelihood of multiple births (30 percent of IVF pregnancies result in multiple births) and possibly even birth defects, because the scientific procedure largely supplants the process of natural selection—in fact, that's the whole idea. The potent steroid hormones used to promote ovulation and/or ripen the egg in the uterus are given at much larger doses than are produced naturally. Although most IVF-conceived children don't suffer any long-term effects, no one really knows the potential long-term consequences of these treatments on either the woman, the child, society, or evolution. But we do know that the *emotional* toll on the couple undergoing IVF is near universal, and often immeasurable.

It was amid all these stresses that Jane first came to see me. We discussed her goals and aspirations, along with where she was in her life at that moment. I challenged her and her husband to consider the questions "Are you in a good place to get pregnant?" and "Is the time right?" While they seemed prepared on several levels—and while it might be true there never really is a perfect time to get pregnant—there seemed to be something else that might be getting in their way. Was Jane really ambivalent about pregnancy, given the pressures of her and Owen's demanding careers? Was she concerned about their lack of a permanent home?

I mentioned to Jane that while she and Owen had a place to live, they weren't "grounded," a helpful state for conception. I reiterated the point: "Isn't it reasonable to assume that a person who doesn't 'nest' is going to struggle with fertility issues, too?" As we delved further, I spoke to Jane about acknowledging certain other rhythms and cycles.

Like many modern women, Jane didn't eat ideally, in a peaceful state of mind and at a table, nor did she rest enough or exercise regularly. She was disconnected from nature, work having surrounded her in environments like offices, gymnasiums, cramped train cars, and overcrowded restaurants. She was a smart woman. She had a tangential awareness of the basic cycles of sleeping and eating but certainly hadn't tried to fit them into her busy life. She even had trouble incorporating her menstrual cycle into her life, always seeing it as a mere inconvenience rather than a natural, life-affirming cycle.

In particular, I encouraged her to honor the day/night cycle and her circadian rhythm. We spoke about going to sleep no later than eleven o'clock; avoiding food after a certain hour, which would be helped by turning in earlier; waking up at sunrise and not sleeping late; and getting adequate sun exposure by going outside more regularly. All this seemed logical, simple, and "natural," so Jane didn't balk.

Then we talked about her work schedule. Jane was intuitively ready to make changes, to make room for a new life. Many women put off conception indefinitely because they claim to have no time, or can't imagine a way to fit children into their hectic schedules. Others give birth, only to run back to work a few short weeks later, leaving their infant in the care of a nanny or a relative. The prevalence of this mindset and its effect even on women who choose the more traditional path is suggestive of a society that has become unhinged from the natural way. Imagine advising the average woman of childbearing age to "settle down, forget about your career and other extraneous pursuits. Enjoy this time in your life." How many women would take this suggestion seriously? Frankly, many would consider it chauvinistic. That's a shame. I don't mean to say a woman should be kept "barefoot and pregnant." I mean to say that *if* you're a woman who would like to have a child, then the best, most skillful, most healthful way to do that is to reconnect with a natural rhythm conducive to conception.

After eighteen months of frustration, Jane was willing to give it a chance. Once she was on a more natural sleep and eating routine, we discussed her beginning to respect a seven-day cycle, including the important day of rest so common in many traditions. The idea of a Sabbath, a departure from regular activities to embrace peace, family, and self-reflection, was a particular challenge for Jane and Owen—as it would be for most professional couples. But I persisted.

I suggested Jane start off her "Sabbath" day with a meal of specially prepared foods, candles, and a fresh bouquet of flowers. These accoutrements make the day feel special and set up a celebratory ritual. I also recommended that on this one day a week, they turn off most electronic devices, including the phone, television, and radio. I asked Jane to consider taking a walk, nothing too physically strenuous, but something that would allow husband and wife to enjoy and connect with nature as well as with each other. This Sabbath day could also include participation in some sort of special activity, such as a casual dinner or afternoon tea with friends.

Once they had embraced the day of rest, I pointed out to Jane the close correlation between the number of days in the lunar and menstrual cycles, highlighting the role of the moon in fertility. I believe that we have devalued this connection, grossly affecting the normal menstrual cycle and thus fertility (as well as another common gynecological "problem," menopause). So I encouraged Jane to set aside time to honor the moon in some way. She could say a special prayer of her own, recite a poem, or simply go outside and feel its presence on a regular basis. But let me be clear. This was not some hippie baying-at-the-moon ritual. In fact, technically, it had nothing to do with the moon per se. The idea here was intended to give Jane a pal-

pable evening reminder of her connection with nature, and to offer
the opportunity for peace and meditation. I also wanted to remind
her that the great and sacred cycles of menstruation and fertility are
fundamental realities of physical life. Understanding and *honoring* the
ways these personal cycles interplay with the greater cycles of our
vast and complex universe is part of our glory, and at the root of our
health. And yet many women have treated the essential cycles of fertility and menstruation disdainfully and with callous disregard. As
Dr. Christiane Northrup has observed, "Nothing in our society, with
the exception of violence and fear, has been more effective in keeping
women in their place than the degradation of the menstrual cycle."[19]
I understand Northrup's use of the word "degradation" to imply the
reduction in status of women in modern society (i.e., a lowering of
their grade/rank/value). I think she selected that word carefully to
impart a negative tone, going so far as to suggest a general hostility and disdain toward women and their natural cycles. The literal
translation—"reducing grade"—clarifies the "second-class citizen-
ship" that women have suffered, which has caused us all, men and
women, to suffer degraded *relationships* and roles in families and in
society as a whole. So, just to make it perfectly clear, this trend does
not bode well for men either.

Jane's journey back into rhythm started out with simple gratitude
for the permission I gave her to indulge in a short, peaceful time alone,
away from her iPhone and the evening news. But looking nightly at
the waxing and waning moon from the window of her home, Jane
eventually began to appreciate how she and her own cycles fit into the
beautiful rhythms of the universe. She began to feel more "open" to
getting pregnant. That's the best way she was able to describe it, and
I understood.

Finally, we discussed seasonal cycles. Was Jane engaging in activities and habits that were seasonally appropriate? Do you? Do you rest

in the winter? Do you revivify outside during the spring? Do you take time to reflect in the fall? I also wanted to know if she was following seasonally appropriate eating habits, another good question to ask yourself. Does your diet consist of oranges in July and blueberries in January, or are you in line with nature's offerings?

As we can all occasionally benefit from a little outside intervention, I suggested to Jane that she might also try some energy work or visit a specialist in Chinese medicine, who could offer the balancing effects of acupuncture and might complement all this attention with a fertility-enhancing remedy or herb that would help her connect to Mother Earth. Finally, for Jane, I specifically recommended Maya abdominal massage, which has been known and practiced for thousands of years by indigenous peoples throughout the world. Maya massage is a noninvasive external massage technique that focuses on the abdomen and pelvis, and is intended to help guide the internal reproductive organs into their proper position while simultaneously relieving tension. Adherents believe that Maya massage improves organ function by releasing physical and emotional congestion and restoring health in the pelvic region. From my experience, the approach is reminiscent of the nurturing quality of a grandmother's touch, and I thought it might be the final piece in helping bring Jane into a more aligned and balanced state.

On some level, eager as she was, I expected Jane to be skeptical of some of my suggested lifestyle changes. Like many of you, she probably thought some were overly simple, New Age-y, or at least unscientific. But she was willing, and she adopted them.

Three months after first visiting my office, Jane was pregnant. Certainly, I don't want to dismiss the contributions of Jane's other doctors, who continued with her regular fertility treatments. But Jane was certain that the key to her conceiving was in realigning herself with nature. Of course, I'm inclined to agree.

22. Do You Observe a Day of Rest Completely Away from Work, Dedicated to Nurturing Yourself and Your Family?

PRACTICAL PRESCRIPTION 3: CELEBRATING A SABBATH

Connecting to a vital source can be as simple as sitting down to a regular weekly meal. In many parts of Europe, the classic Sunday dining experience includes church services in the morning, followed by a leisurely afternoon meal with family and friends that often extends into early evening. Observant Jews all over the world do this on Saturday, the Shabbos. People look forward to this Sabbath day; there's no work, no distractions. Children play and adults socialize, read, pray, reflect, or just hang out. It's only natural that after a period of work, we need a period of balanced rest. Long ago, we discovered that a field must lie fallow once every seven years in order to produce the most abundant fruit. We allow our best academic minds a year off—a sabbatical—to study and reflect every seven years, too. In many religious traditions, including the Judeo-Christian, our creator worked tirelessly to make the world—then rested, and requested that we follow suit.

But you needn't necessarily add a religious overtone to a classic day of rest. Instead you could think of it as a day to yourself and your thoughts, to mark the culmination of the weekly cycle, in every sense of the word. A Sabbath day is an opportunity to renew and reconstitute, to reconnect with each other, with nature, with the life force, and to help you prepare for the coming week's challenges. I urge you to try it. I think it's a very healthy tradition.

QUESTIONS FOR FURTHER REFLECTION

23. Do You Feel a Strong Connection to and Appreciation for Your Home and Your Environment?

24. Do You Take Time to Relax with Activities That Require Abandon or Absorption or Play?

25. Do You Maintain Physically Challenging Goals?

Think back to your childhood. Would any one of these questions even cross your mind? Of course not. When you're a child, you simply live your life in the moment. You find yourself connected to nature without a care, absorbed in play and pushing your limits, physically and in every other way. Indeed, you're quite *alive* as a child, and therefore quite healthy. So what happened between then and now? That's a complicated question, but it doesn't really matter. What matters is whether you can find your way back, rekindling the fire of freedom you experienced then, so you can reclaim much of your vitality in the *now*. Not sure you have the tools to do it? Just look at a photo of yourself when you were three.

RECLAIMING CONTROL:
READYING YOURSELF FOR CHANGE

AUTOBIOGRAPHY IN FIVE SHORT CHAPTERS

CHAPTER ONE
I walk down the street.
There is a deep hole in the sidewalk
I fall in.
I am lost . . . I am hopeless.
It isn't my fault.
It takes forever to find a way out.

CHAPTER TWO
I walk down the same street.
There is a deep hole in the sidewalk.
I pretend I don't see it.
I fall in again.
I can't believe I'm in the same place.
But it isn't my fault.
It still takes a long time to get out.

CHAPTER THREE
I walk down the same street.
There is a deep hole in the sidewalk.
I see it is there.
I still fall in . . . it's a habit.
My eyes are open.
I know where I am.
It is MY fault.
I get out immediately.

CHAPTER FOUR
I walk down the same street.
There is a deep hole in the sidewalk.
I walk around it.

CHAPTER FIVE
I walk down another street.

—Portia Nelson[1]

26. Do You Believe It's Possible to Change?

I think by now you're starting to understand and value a more holistic approach to healing what ails you. And by now, you're beginning to take stock of your overall health, according to our new, wider, and wiser definition. Now I want to prepare you to make some real changes. In this chapter, I want to give you some practical, but no less inspirational, tools to take the first steps and address the most common obstacles to getting started: denial, resistance, and fear, the things we feel most often when we're facing change—even positive change.

Albert Einstein writes, "The world as we have created it is a process of our thinking. We cannot change the world without changing our thinking."[2] So, first and foremost, if you're going to change, you've got to *believe* you can change. And you've got to take *responsibility*. This means, literally, the ability to respond. You must summon your courage and remember that you have the ability to respond right now. In your choices. In your beliefs. In your actions. The person who falls in the proverbial hole in the above poem might at first believe "it's not my fault." But where does such lack of responsibility get you? Out of the hole and back into the light? Sure, maybe someone else shouldn't have left that hole there for someone to fall in. Maybe someone even pushed that poor, defenseless person into that hole. But what does it matter? No amount of righteous indignation will get your butt back on the street. You and only you have the ability to respond right now. To pull yourself up and out.

The conventional medical system doesn't allow for that kind of self-motivated boost. It, along with the rest of Western culture, has taught us to be helpless. This "learned helplessness" comes when we humans or other animals undergo an unpleasant event or a series of events that we perceive, either rightly or wrongly, that we can do nothing about. Take an elephant getting shocked by a trainer's electric prod. At first, she tries to resist. But she soon—often *very* soon—discovers that she can't get free of her restraints to avoid the prod. After a short while, she gives up trying. She will just lie down and take the shock, over and over. She might *hope* that bad things will stop happening to her, but she will not *believe* she can do anything about them—so she will not even try. This is one of the reasons that despite how powerful they can be, elephants in captivity don't require massive chains to keep them docile. A simple string will work. Having been conditioned for learned helplessness, as soon as the elephant senses the slightest resistance on her hoof, she will stop trying to pull herself free.

Since the 1960s, countless experiments with rats, mice, dogs, and even human test subjects have proved that learned helplessness happens, and it hurts our chances for improving our current conditions. So if you *believe* that there's nothing you can do about your health condition, then you won't do anything about your health condition. It's insidious, and it's a slippery slope as well. Initially you take less care of yourself, but eventually you wind up actively self-destructive. I don't want to come off sounding judgmental or insensitive, but this is the truth, and what you're likely to see when you really look in the mirror. Allowing yourself to fall victim to learned helplessness hurts your chances for better health. Sure, the whole rest of the herd might be doing the same thing, but there's no safety in those numbers.

Correcting for all other contributing factors, people who feel helpless about their medical conditions feel worse, do worse, and die faster.[3] It's a proven fact. And it's not just a question of some self-fulfilling psychological prophecy—people with learned helplessness face worse health outcomes because their physical conditions deteriorate faster when they are pessimistic about their ability to control their health. There's intriguing science, for example, showing that tumors grow faster in animals that have been conditioned for learned helplessness.[4, 5]

So, ask yourself, Do I believe it's possible to change? Deep down inside, I think you do. But if you've been confronted with challenges that were hard to overcome, you might be pessimistic. If so, stay with me. On the other side, if you're already certain that change is possible, then the next step for you will be to make changes happen in your own life. And that isn't easy either. So where do you go from here?

The next thing to do is to be honest with yourself. This is not the same as evaluating and judging, but rather just taking a good look, and working on clearly understanding how you got to where you are. There's no need to place blame. Instead, this is akin to taking an inventory, taking stock in your current predicament so that you can clearly identify what's contributing to your situation.

When you do this, you're likely to notice many things, including some flaws and bad habits. Perhaps the most important one of these, however, is any tendency you might have to accept someone else's measure of your value. The labels that we tend to place on ourselves as a result are most certainly a reflection of our acceptance of someone else's rules. These can be important, but they're often not completely accurate, and sometimes they're intentionally repressive. This is why it's so important to assess the situation for yourself. The 77 Skillful Questions become a tool you can use for this purpose—to take inventory. With these skillful questions guiding you, you'll be able to take a good survey of your situation and see where the opportunities for improvement—i.e., alignment—exist.

So examine the question again: Isn't real change possible? What do you think now? What's holding you back from accepting responsibility to change yourself? Can you at least give it a chance? If so, you are ready to take the next step: making the change happen in your own life.

A GOOD LOOK IN THE MIRROR

Of course that's easier said than done. Anyone who's ever tried to quit smoking or lose weight knows that these habits "do not go gentle into that good night." Similarly, the nihilism about change can become a habit. So where do habits come from? And how do we finally overcome them?

Often, we're unaware that we're getting into a certain habit. Unskillful habits like poor eating and sloth tend to develop gradually, silently, without our intention. In some ways, this makes them more insidious and powerful once they're set. Speaking as a doctor as well as a fellow human being, I can tell you that ingrained habits are very hard to reverse, but by no means impossible. It's just that, as Einstein so presciently observed, we have to change the *thinking* that led to the habit, the thought processes or lack thereof that ultimately sustain the habit. As an example, millions of people who go on diets every year lose weight—sometimes a lot. Yet a full 95 percent of them gain all or most of the weight back within a year.[6] Why? Without shifting our *thinking,* we can't expect a durable change in our behavior.

Luckily, there's good news on this front. Strong *motivators,* both positive (such as rewards) and negative (such as a trauma or chronic illness), can help break even the most deeply ingrained habits. We can use external motivators to help us change habits. We can think about *why* we want to get better, and keep our eyes on that prize. Perhaps we can visualize lifting our grandchildren for the first time in years. Or breaking the ribbon at the end of a 5K run. On the other side of the equation, we can use a milestone of crisis—such as receiving a diabetes diagnosis—as a motivator for growth and development. True, crises almost never come at a convenient time, and the pain and anxiety they produce sometimes lead us to seek an immediate, Band-Aid solution from outside ourselves—some drug or other treatment. Sometimes this is important or even necessary, just to get us through. But it's short-lived and, in the end, not enough. However, if we can remain balanced, present, and focused for long enough, we might get a glimpse of something more meaningful on a deeper level, something that helps us make the change we know we need.

But you don't have to promise yourself a trip to Hawaii for losing fifty pounds—and you don't have to wait for your first heart attack to break unskillful and unhealthy habits. You just have to be willing to do a careful and honest self-inventory.

On both personal and professional levels, I've found that sincere self-reflection is one of the most important and skillful steps for modifying behavior. Like all animals, we eat, sleep, and reproduce; we experience sensations, emotions, and perceptions; and we take in knowledge about our external world. Unlike other animals, however, we possess this remarkable capacity for self-reflection. Zen Buddhism refers to our facility for looking in the mirror, or more accurately for self-knowledge, as the "distinguishing mark of authentic human existence."[7]

You don't have to be a Zen master to do this. It's easier than it sounds. Find a quiet place and consider your health situation, your body, your feelings, your sense of balance and peace—or lack thereof. Be honest. Ask meaningful questions. Am I feeling well? Am I eating well? Am I sleeping well? Am I too reliant on drugs? Am I feeling like a victim? Am I balanced? What hole do I keep falling into—and why? The trick here is not to coddle yourself, not to make excuses and justifications, but to find places for improvement. Then work on gathering the courage to change. You should rely here not on the "experts"—not even on me!—but on your own instincts and judgments about where you are and where you need to go. So you don't feel overwhelmed, you can focus on one health aspect at a time—the most important thing first.

WHAT WOULD HAPPEN IF PATIENTS STOPPED PLAYING THE VICTIM?

This self-reflection and self-inventory is a far cry from our current way of thinking about our health. Our whole health care system is based on the notion of an unwise patient playing victim to an "expert" doctor. "Help me," the patient says. "I'm broken." There's very little room in this equation for responsibility. The patient isn't looking in the mirror but at his doctor. Yet the vast majority of chronic health problems we face—the Big 8 and the top killers—are profoundly subject to our own intervention. By and large, they are diseases of lifestyle, not genetics. When genetics does play a part by loading the gun, it's still our lifestyle choices that pull the trigger. Meaning we got ourselves into this unskillful mess, and we can get ourselves out by looking in the mirror and acting responsibly. By making different decisions along the way, starting today. Change won't happen passively. It won't happen by osmosis, and it won't fall from the sky. It's in your hands. It certainly won't happen if you keep avoiding your eyes in that mirror. I know it might feel painful even to think about it, but I promise you that you'll feel better for it. Certainly, you need some courage to do this. But let's first look at why you might be feeling uneasy about embracing a new course.

OUR HERD MENTALITY

How do we get in these holes, health-wise and otherwise? Why are we resistant to looking in the mirror? One of the big obstacles to our moving toward extraordinary health—to change in general—is our resistance to autonomy, true freedom from outside influence. It's a real paradox, because we Americans have come to think of ourselves as rebels, as archetypal rugged individualists who are entirely self-reliant. But if you look around, don't you find we're really more like a bunch of proverbial lemmings, lining up on the cliff, ready to follow our fellows into the briny deep? Do you think that's too extreme? That it doesn't refer to you? Well, let's think about it.

We certainly agree that we have this tendency to resist change. And I think it's reasonable to assert that's mainly because so many of us are overly concerned with what others—our parents, our children, our neighbor, our spouse, our doctor—might say. As a culture, we're trained to avoid appearing too special, too novel, too different from the crowd. Yes, our society tolerates a certain amount of individuality and even iconoclasm—especially among celebrities. Lady Gaga can get away with dressing in a meat costume or arriving on the red carpet curled up in a giant egg—she can even make millions of dollars while doing it. But try showing up at your bank that way, or your office, and see what happens. You'll find that the dominant culture treats most eccentricity (defined as standing out from the crowd) censoriously at best. This is particularly true when we violate social mores or somehow seem to challenge venerable institutions, such as the Catholic Church—or the standard American diet.

There are good reasons for this in evolutionary adaptation: there is often safety in numbers. Tribalism itself has great evolutionary advantages, not to mention that it makes life more pleasant as a rule. We need to band together to survive, and we generally enjoy each other's company—at least those who are like "us," not like "them" over there. And surely much moral good has come from agreeing together, more or less, on codes of behavior that serve the individual *and* collective good—though we know that variously interpreting and misinterpreting these codes causes unending strife as well.

In general, humans have a herd mentality, not unlike that of other animals, and this herd mentality originates in fear. In nature, a wildebeest avoiding a lion best illustrates the nature of this herd behavior. Each member of the herd minimizes the danger to *itself* by choosing the location and action/behavior that is as close to the center of the *group* as possible (no wildebeest goes off and lives by his own devices as a rugged *individual,* because he would be the lion's first meal).

Experts and the media offer the concept of herd mentality as an explanation for phenomena where large numbers of people act in the same way at the same time, such as in the case of the rioting and looting that overcame London in 2011. In his 1896 work *The Crowd: A Study of the Popular Mind,* social psychologist Gustave Le Bon set the stage for our understanding of human herd mentality: "Crowds, after a period of excitement, enter upon a purely automatic and unconscious state, in which they are guided by suggestion."[8] This essentially means the group drives the individuals.

Since Le Bon's seminal work, more modern studies have striven to debunk his theory, arguing vehemently for the idea that crowds are just groups of individuals acting in their own best interest. Evolutionary biologist W. D. Hamilton writes about this subject in a famous paper, "Geometry for the Selfish Herd," which was published more than three decades ago in the *Journal of Theoretical Biology*. Hamilton writes that while a herd appears to move and act as one, much like a flock of birds, its pattern actually emerges from the paradoxically uncoordinated behavior of individuals seeking self-preservation. Individually, humans also naturally protect themselves in this way.[9]

But most sociologists who study crowds still argue that "group identity is a precondition for a riot: People will only riot when they think their actions are aligned with the worldview of the group as a whole."[10] In other words, assuming you are compelled to act contrary to the usual norm—say, by breaking a window with a brick—you, as an individual actor, feel you can get away with this only as long as you're amid a large crowd where others are also acting unusually. In other words, you're still relying on the implicit sanctioning by the local "masses" for your individual behavior.

Not that all herd behavior is violent or aggressive. Some herd behavior has innocuous consequences, such as whole groups of high school juniors wearing skinny jeans, thousands mass-Tweeting after the debut of the new season of *The Walking Dead*, or fans of a sports team jeering the opposing team at a game. However, too often the herd mind-set leads to the excesses of widespread rioting. Why do we go with the crowd, even when we know it might not be in our best interest? As Professor Louis René Beres argues in a recent *Washington Times* editorial, more than almost anything else, human beings need to belong:

> *In all cases the individual person feels empty and insignificant*
> *apart from his/her membership in the herd. Sometimes that herd*

is the state. Sometimes it is the tribe. Sometimes it is the faith.
Sometimes it is the "liberation" or "revolutionary" organization.
But whatever the particular herd of the moment, it is the persistent
craving for membership that brings the terrible downfall of individual
responsibility and the terrifying triumph of the collective will.[11]

The key here is "the terrible downfall of individual responsibility." This makes me think of the rise of the Nazi Party in the 1930s. We'd like to think a Holocaust could never happen again, but couldn't it? How were the regular people of Germany different from us now? And what happens when followers are misled by leaders who are themselves misguided? Or when there are no discernible leaders besides the mob itself? That's a good way of looking at many of the decisions we make daily based on what the group around us is doing, even when their behaviors or beliefs violate our own instincts. Looking at each other instead of in the mirror, following the crowd, we keep falling into the same holes—and we keep declaring, "It isn't my fault." It takes us a long time to get out.

What does all this have to do with health? To find extraordinary health, you have to be willing to buck the herd, seek your own truths, and avoid the typical traps into which the masses fall on their run across the landscape. Look *inside*, not out.

27. Are You Happy with Your Body and At or Near a Healthy Body Weight?

STARTING SIMPLY

Let's begin with the basics: body weight and diet. I start with these because I know they're on your mind—and in your mirror.

There's a lot of advice out there about something called your ideal body weight (IBW). You might remember those old actuarial charts from insurance companies, where you cross-referenced your height, age, and gender to find out what you should weigh. Ever since the 1950s, life insurance companies began basing that "should" on the weight above which people of your gender and frame size began to have health problems—like *death*, the ultimate health problem—that cost them (the company) cold, hard cash. If they could keep you at or below that IBW, they could keep from paying out big benefits to your family. Meantime, if your weight fell above the IBW, they could charge you a higher premium. There's some truth to this. That extra weight really does cost the system more money in health care costs.

Nowadays, there are more precise statistics backed by the medical establishment, basically determined in the same way as the insurance companies did years ago: What are the weights at which people begin to suffer high blood pressure, heart disease, osteoarthritis, diabetes, cancer, and so forth, the so-called comorbid conditions associated with excess weight? Online IBW calculators abound if you want to see where you fall. However, be warned that many of these formulas are out of date, some are contradictory, and several are awfully confusing. (Do you really have to measure your elbow breadth to figure out your frame size?)

Note that IBW is closely related to another measurement you've probably heard of from your doctor or your insurance company: body mass index (BMI). BMI approximates the percentage of body fat on your frame. Again, you can consult a multitude of online tools to help you calculate this ratio if you want to see where you fit or don't fit.

I don't reject the notions of IBW or BMI from a statistical standpoint. The truth is, you're far less likely to encounter significant chronic health problems if you're carrying less weight—specifically, less fat—on your frame. These formulas can also be helpful from a diagnostic viewpoint. They remind us that obesity (BMI greater than $30kg/m^2$) and overweight (BMI in the range of 25 to $30kg/m^2$) are clinical epidemics in the United States, with about 56 percent of the population suffering.[12]

But I'm going to keep it much simpler for you, with no charts, measurements, or math. Just look in the mirror. How do you look? Get naked. How do you feel? Take a walk. How does your body perform? Does your intuition tell you that your weight and/or percentage of fat is not "ideal" for you? Too much? Too little? If so, are you ready to make a change? Are you prepared to start doing a few critical things differently?

It would be fantastic to feel and look better. Good for your confidence. Your job. Your sex life. For keeping up with your kids. For your tennis game. Across-the-board good. And good on a much deeper level, too. Good for your health and your future.

But I'm living in the real world with you. I'm not going to ask you to strive for a mathematical ideal. Truth is, very few of us can or will achieve that. I'm going to ask you to think about it. Get a feel for where you are. Use your intuition to determine how far off you are from the "ideal," and be willing to start a process that moves you in the right direction. The most important part is honestly assessing your body and committing to making some changes if necessary (if you're still reading this book, I'm willing to bet some changes are necessary and you're willing to make them).

So what's the slow medicine prescription for weight loss? Do you need to spend hundreds on materials? Do you need to study chemistry and biology, hire a nutritionist? No. It's super-simple, actually: Chuck the cans, bags, and boxes and eat whole foods (things with one ingredient), with a preponderance of fruits and vegetables. Cut down on excessive meat, fat, and protein. Yes, there's more to know, but starting here gets you 90 percent of the way. Oh, and start eating a little less and moving a little more. That's it. With that simple a program, you'll be on your way to extraordinary wellness.

To remind you, though, you have to *make* a change. And to do that, you have to believe you can—and should—make a change. Your best tools here are your intuition and your mirror—not your peers in the herd. If you look around at your family, friends, coworkers, and fellow citizens at the mall, you're going to conclude, logically, that your weight is "average" and therefore okay. But it might not be. As you're standing there, look carefully at your waistline. Feel for excess "baggage" around your middle, where it can be the most unhealthy. How do you feel when you're naked? Ask yourself whether you still fit into the pants you wore when you were twenty-two? Twenty-five? Thirty-five? This is the objective reality that should prompt you to action.

28. Do You Maintain a Skillful Diet, Low in Processed and Refined Foods and Animal Products and High in Fresh, Seasonal Fruits and Vegetables?

THE HUNGRY HERD

Putting down the junk food isn't easy. Let's talk about why. The fact is, you might have a nasty habit, and you might be a little out of control when it comes to what you eat and how much you eat. We all know the herd has taken us to the trough of unskillful eating, meal after meal, snack after snack, treat after treat, until we've become less healthy than past generations, despite—and sometimes because of—the enormous "advances" we've made in food science and medicine. On our continent, obesity is now the second leading cause of death.[13] For a decade or more, for the first time in history, there are just as many overweight people (1.2 billion) as there are underfed people in the world.[14] If we don't step away from the feeding trough, in a little more than a decade, 75 percent of North Americans will be overweight. We might all be in this (sinking) boat together, but that's cold comfort. All this excess weight:

- raises your blood cholesterol and triglyceride levels
- lowers your HDL ("good") cholesterol
- raises your blood pressure levels
- increases your heart attack risk
- increases your diabetes risk
- increases your osteoarthritis risk
- saps your energy
- interferes with your sleep
- contributes to your depression, guilt, and shame

If you're even mildly overweight, your chance of getting diabetes doubles. If you're obese, the chance triples, which explains why more than twenty-one million people in the United States have diabetes and forty-one million more have prediabetes.[15] Type 2 diabetes and overweight are twin-sister conditions: when one increases, so does the other.

Here's where we must look at the herd around us. The cultural element weighs heavily, pun intended. It starts with our first herd—our family. We think of diabetes and obesity as genetic: my mama had it, so I have it. But that's an issue not of genes, but plates. Your mama teaches you how to eat. You and your mama are sitting around the same table, making the same food choices.

As a society (a big herd), we're seeing some pretty alarming trends. We're consuming five hundred to eight hundred more calories per day than we did in the 1970s (about a 24.5 percent increase). Generally deadly refined grains, sugars, fats, and oils make up more than 90 percent of these extra calories.[16] Restaurant portion sizes have at least doubled—and in most cases *quadrupled*—from their 1950s equivalents, when the *Happy Days* gang, Richie and Potsie and Ralph, went to the diner once or twice a week (after burning all those calories necking with girls). French fry portions nearly quadrupled from the average portion of 2.4 ounces at Al's. A hamburger patty has tripled from the 3.9 ounces in the 1950s to the common 12 ounces at restaurants today. The average pasta serving has doubled, as have muffin sizes. And a chocolate bar, which averaged one ounce when Mrs. Cunningham served it to Joanie in the 1950s, is now on average up to *eight times bigger!*[17] Meantime, are we exercising eight times more? You know the answer to that.

In the United States and Europe, people consume an average of about 3,550 calories daily. By contrast, people in Asia consume on average 2,648 calories daily. The diet in these Eastern countries seems to rely mostly on whole grains and vegetables, with far less meat than we consume. In Western countries, meats and fats make up a significantly larger portion of the diet.[18] Which culture do you suppose is fatter, less healthy, and unhappier? It probably won't surprise you to know that as Western influences like McDonald's settle firmly in the East, people there have begun to look and feel more like us. What a terrible legacy.

What led us to this? What leads us to make these kinds of choices? Is there some other hollowness we're trying to fill besides our stomachs? I believe there is. We as individuals are no longer eating strictly from physical hunger. And we as a culture certainly don't have to worry about famine and starvation anymore. Our problems have a lot more to do with excess than lack. So what's behind the decisions we're making? Next time you want to reach for the doughnut or cookie, try employing a little more common sense and wisdom. Use your mirror. Ask yourself, Am I really hungry? Or am I feeling useless in my career? Am I feeling unloved and unattractive to the world? Am I feeling unfulfilled in my creative endeavors? Am I trying to build a barrier between an uncaring world and my sensitive self? Am I, in short, treating feelings with food? None of these questions is pleasant, I know. But neither are illness and needless early death after years of pain. Many of these questions and their answers fall under the umbrella of a syndrome called emotional eating. Overeating has long been associated with depression, anxiety, loneliness, boredom, anger, low self-esteem, and a host of other emotional states, in addition to all its negative effects on the physical body. I understand how tempting it is to keep denying and resisting the change. But I also know how unskillful that is.

Let me be clear: it's not fair to oversimplify the challenges you face, or to categorize you in any way. I'm not judging you, but asking you to look deeper into the personal and cultural factors that might have led to the health state you're in—and the one you want to be free of. With the right questions, I hope you might finally understand the emotional elements that influence you and your health choices, and gain the clarity you need to take the necessary steps to becoming healthier. I'm saying that something else out there will make you feel more full than a pint of rum raisin ice cream. It's not for me to dictate what exactly that something is, but I think that the vast majority of times, it has a lot less to do with physical hunger than with the spiritual, emotional, and soul-level hunger I discussed earlier. When you learn to properly care for and feed those aspects of your life, your stomach tends to stop grumbling.

All of this makes me think of my patient Barry. He told me he had been successful twenty-one times in losing weight, a remarkable achievement, on the one hand. Unfortunately, he also relapsed twenty-one times, so typical of the roller-coaster ride of dieting. But Barry was no slouch. He was intelligent and well-meaning, a wonderful man. He was also very well versed in the lingo of dieting. In fact, he could recite the ten most popular diets off the top of his head, with all the details and instructions as clear as I've ever heard them. He was not failing for lack of information or intention. He was simply in a rut, familiar to so many. Like others, he also subscribed to the simple formula of calories in/calories out. So he exercised a great deal. But he was still overweight and suffering from it. He was working hard and getting nowhere. When I met him, he was very down, experiencing even more frustration and depression as a result of all his "failures." This only contributed to his pain. Like most, Barry was barking up the wrong tree—constantly looking for answers and the next great approach that would finally solve his problem.

I sat Barry down, as I do with all my patients, and asked him to identify all the pieces of his health puzzle, from his physical symptoms to his feelings about his relationships and work. I asked him a question that simply blew him away: I said, if I were a magician and could simply restore your weight (and resolve every ailment and problem you're experiencing), what would you *do* with your newfound health? What would you do with your life? In other words: Where are you going? What's your purpose? After he wiped the tears from his eyes, he knew what he needed to do. He needed to get his life in order. Not his weight. His life.

Several months later, with the puzzle pieces in place, Barry was a new man. It wasn't the result of a newfangled diet. It was the guidance within that steered him to fulfill his purpose, a real purpose. Meaning returned to his life and he was back on track. Months after that, without nearly the effort he had put in previously, he shed the weight. He has never looked back.

You, too, could follow the crowds to the buffet, or you could turn to look inside, the way your instinct tells you that you must. You know something needs to change. But to ready yourself for real change in your health, you've got to buck that crowd that has given you permission to overeat and eat the wrong foods. The herd of your family. The herd of the Wal-Mart culture. The herd of TV ads that declare "I'm lovin' it!" Loving what? Diabetes? Heart attacks? Early death? No—loving the taste. The mouth feel. The surge you feel when you first ingest that kind of stuff. It's no accident: a lot of careful planning and high-tech science makes sure you feel a strong kind of high when you eat junk food. The idea is simple: junk food *is* a drug. I don't mean metaphorically, but *literally*. Sugar and fat and artificial chemicals work the same way on brain chemistry as drugs like cocaine do. Pile in that mac and cheese, full of butter, salt, and highly processed white flour, and the brain very soon gets a boost of dopamine. Of course we all know it crashes soon after, then sends us in search of another quick fix. Studies show we'll ignore almost all other impulses in order to get it. We feel *secure* somehow, once we get this junk food fix, and we really suffer without it.

There's a reason they call it comfort food; things that feel good (like sex and eating) are *supposed* to be good for us, supposed to ensure we survive and reproduce. But science has short-circuited this process. So now our brains interpret the feeling we get from sugar, fat, and other junk as security to counter our inherited fear of famine. But of course, we're far from famished.

Contributing to our chemical quest for that quick fix is a pervasive psychological problem: the constant peer pressure we undergo from family, friends, and the media. We hear constant enabling messages: *Have another drink. Splurge a little. You deserve a treat.* This pattern often begins with our mothers, I'm afraid to say. What does love smell like? Isn't it Mom's chocolate chip cookies, or her gravy, or her [insert your mother's specialty here]? Is it any wonder so many of us are emotional eaters who confuse food with feelings?

I love food, but food is not love. No amount of pepperoni pizza will make up for a dearth of love in your life. In fact, the pizza is much more likely to make you feel further depressed.

Try whole foods. Prepare them yourself, or with loved ones, carefully, lovingly, and slowly. Celebrate the meals. Feel grateful for the bounty. Fill yourself throughout your life with all the joys of living, whenever you can. Don't look to fulfill your spiritual and emotional hunger with fat, protein, and sugar. There's no love at the bottom of a bucket of chicken—just grease and regret.

DENIAL

When the solutions are so simple, why is it so hard to make real changes? One reason is that old enemy of change: denial. We'd like to pretend that everything's okay. It's a built-in defense mechanism.

In his transcendent poem "The Marriage of Heaven and Hell," William Blake writes, "If the fool would persist in his folly he would become wise." For many of us, the paradigm shift toward wisdom never occurs, and we persist in our folly until we fall into the hole again and again, never choosing to walk down the other street instead.

The struggle to learn from our experiences seems to be the root cause of a broad range of problems afflicting society, from substance abuse and obesity to the widespread mistreatment of the planet and exploitation of its resources. Think about it: Don't you think it's a good bet that most hardened alcoholics, drug addicts, bullies, and polluters are aware of the harm their actions are causing? Many subtler forms of self-destructive behavior also go on despite a general recognition of their damaging effects. Yet we persist in hurting others and ourselves despite the consequences. Why? Why do so many of us deny the problem and fail to alter our behavior? Why do we fear the mirror?

Maybe it's because we know on some level that looking in our own eyes will reveal that we've made some unskillful choices—that it's all on us. We can't really blame "Mom" or "society" or "genetics" or "the media." And maybe it's because we know that real change demands continuous hard work.

We can think of this as our herd's collective tendency toward languor and laziness when it comes to changing behavior. We're biologically hardwired to seek maximum benefits from minimal effort. So perhaps our resistance might be the natural response to the realization of how hard the work is. Why bother? It's so much easier to turn on the TV and settle in with a box of cookies.

This form of laziness often manifests as denial. We *justify*. We talk ourselves into believing that it's okay to maintain the status quo. This is especially true when we look around and see most everyone else doing the same things we are. Laziness might also be a reflection of a deep-seated feeling we have that fundamentally we're not worthy of a better life. We look in the mirror and we see a lost cause, and a cause unworthy of saving. Either way, we experience a self-fulfilling prophecy as our unskillful behavior and unhealthy choices continue to contribute to our low self-esteem and worsening health, and so on in a downward spiral.

Furthering this challenge is that as we lose faith in our ability to take care of ourselves, as we continue to consider ourselves unworthy of real health, we keep looking elsewhere—to the herd and its leaders—for solutions.

Meantime, we keep hiding in our holes. Even when well-meaning doctors try to help us ask the right questions—How much do you drink? Are you taking your medicine? Are you engaging in risky sexual behavior?—we find ourselves embarrassed by the questions and ashamed at the answers we're hiding. It's profoundly paradoxical that we approach our doctors as victims incapable of saving ourselves, but at the same time, we lie through our teeth to them! Or at least we regularly omit certain facts, concoct stories, and shade the truth to make our behavior seem more acceptable. Patients *routinely* lie to their doctors about whether they're taking their medications, understate how much they eat, overstate how much they exercise, feign illnesses to get appointments faster, and ask their doctors to hide information from their insurance companies.[19]

Why do we do this? Because our intuition tells us that we're making unskillful choices. We'd rather deny them than change them.

In fact, denial seems to be the normal state of affairs in our modern society. We deny everything: our finances, health, relationships, habitat destruction, disease, and even the fact of death. We deny problems outright, look for scapegoats, replace uncomfortable emotions or feelings with "appropriate" ones (this is called reaction formation), project our anxieties onto someone or something else (displacement), and/or generally shut out information (suppression) when we find it inconvenient or distasteful.

There's a second interesting paradox at work. While we frequently deny certain things about ourselves, we can deny them only once we have, on some level, recognized and acknowledged them. If you have chest pain every time you walk up a hill, for example, you're *aware* of your condition. But if you choose to ignore it, if you don't share this information and seek solutions, you're denying its existence, at your peril.

Or, when we do finally recognize something, too often we choose to ignore the implications. "Sure, I'm a hundred pounds overweight, but otherwise, I'm healthy." "Yeah, my wife and I don't talk anymore, but that's just the way it goes in a marriage." Perhaps this happens to us when we feel helpless to solve big problems. In times of war and repression, entire communities can become incapacitated by denial. For many years, German Jews closed their eyes to the looming threat of Nazism because they convinced themselves that as loyal and assimilated citizens they were safe. Not to mention the denial on behalf of the non-Jews: What did they think all those trains and smokestacks were for? Did they really think all the Jews, Catholics, Gypsies, and homosexuals were away at summer camp?

Sometimes denial serves a purpose. Because our minds can't possibly attend to everything in our inner and outer worlds, denial of certain conditions and situations helps us focus on our immediate needs. Some people use denial as a coping strategy, and it might even keep them temporarily sane. However, when the issues that lead to denial become recurrent or habitual, then denial becomes an albatross. In my medical practice, I often see heart patients deny that they're feeling lousy, sometimes with serious medical consequences. Such denial, some research has shown, may be a more powerful predictor of heart attacks than familiar risk factors such as smoking, high blood pressure, and diabetes.[20]

Look—if a friend were talking to you about her health, and it emerged that she had serious, chronic issues, would you encourage her to deny them? "Don't worry, Sue. It's just heart disease. Why don't you just ignore it!" Of course you wouldn't. So why don't you deal with your own chronic conditions with the same clarity of understanding, the same respect and attention?

29. Is Your Water Intake Adequate?

Feel like you don't have the energy to face that truth? Too tired to tackle real health change—or any change for that matter? Well, let me shift gears and relieve you of the mounting pressure you might be feeling and return to something much less provocative. Part of the "laziness" that gets in the way of change could be physiological. It

might sound overly simple and even silly, but if you want to be ready
to make a real change in your health, you've got to consider whether
you're hydrated for it. The body is between 60 and 70 percent water
by mass, and water is necessary for every vital organ and process. It
flushes out toxins, it lubricates joints, it carries nutrients to cells, and it
helps the blood flow. Of particular interest to us is how water can help
ease inflammation, the issue at the root of the Big 8.

Yet, as a nation—perhaps as a species—we're chronically dehy-
drated. We lose water constantly through our breath, our sweat, and
our bathroom functions. And we need more water now than ever, to
dilute the load of salts and chemicals we consume. So this one's very
simple: you must replenish those fluids. You've all heard that you should
drink eight eight-ounce glasses of water per day. Recently, there's been
some backlash against that advice, because it's not necessarily supported by hard science. But good sources such as the Mayo Clinic and
the Institute of Medicine recommend that men in temperate climate
zones drink about thirteen eight-ounce glasses a day, women about
nine eight-ounce glasses a day.[21] My advice is similar, but I'd like to
provide you with a simple suggestion for ensuring you're getting close
to the amount you need based on your weight. Drink enough so that
you pee every two or three hours during the day. Your pee should be
light-colored and clear. In all likelihood that will require at least eight
glasses a day, so starting there makes sense after all. Obviously, if you're
exercising and sweating a lot, or if it's particularly hot and humid, you're
going to need more water. And when I say water, I mean water—not
soda, not diet soda, coffee, milk, or fruit juice. A little tea is okay if you
want some extra flavor. An occasional glass of wine with dinner is okay,
too. But generally, when you think "drink," think water.

Proper hydration will help you look and feel better. It makes the
skin less dry. It prevents headaches and cramps. It will grease your
rusty wheels and get you ready for real change. And in the scheme

of things it's simple. When do I water my garden? I make sure my plants get the water they need at all times. I'll wait while you pour yourself a glass.

30. Do You Stretch Regularly?

In the same way that you would stretch before a bout of physical activity, you should prepare to get ready for the stresses of the average day. Just as a cat or dog does first thing in the morning, you should give your major muscle groups a good stretch when you wake up, or after long periods of inactivity, such as when you've been sitting in front of a laptop for hours. It feels good and it's good for you: stretching helps with flexibility, range of motion, stress relief, back pain, posture, coordination, blood flow, and overall energy. It might even prevent strains and other injuries.[22] On another level, think of the physical stretching of your muscles as preparation for "stretching" yourself toward change in your life.

There are lots of good resources online and in the bookstore to help you with a stretching routine, but much of it is just common sense. A few suggestions, though:

1. Stretching should push (and pull) your muscles to their natural limits, but it should not hurt. If you're feeling pain, dial it back. Slowly increase your stretches over time to increase flexibility and range of motion.

2. For general purposes (not for specific sports performance or enhancement), stretching should be *static,* not *ballistic.* This means you shouldn't "bounce" the muscles, but rather slowly and steadily stretch them. Reach forward until you feel

the tension in your muscle, then hold that stretch for a few seconds. If you're training for soccer or some other athletic activity, consider more *dynamic* stretching, and consider a professional trainer to help you avoid injuries. Remember, stiffness in the body is often a consequence of a rigid mind. Therefore, stretch your mind, too, daily. Learn new things. Remind yourself to consider new possibilities regularly and reach out.

31. Have You Let Go of Fear in Your Life?

FINDING THE PATH AWAY FROM FEAR

Despite the great simplicity of the questions in this chapter, there are reasons that so few of us practice them. Learning to live skill-fully, for all its benefits, can be scary. Asking yourself deep questions about the quality of your life and your potential futures, good and bad, can be particularly frightening. In fact, I've found that fear is at the heart of many of my patients' real health challenges. The good news is, you can work on alleviating fear, starting with the fear of change, and separate yourself from the herd on its way to slaughter.

Fear is a powerful force in the way of our getting better. A culture that's all about following the herd, a medical system that encourages us to come to "expert" doctors as "victims," a system that conditions us to expect quick solutions to difficult problems, a society that doesn't believe we can learn much from challenges, a culture overreli-ant on technology and the latest advancements—all of that's a recipe for hopelessness in the face of chronic health difficulties. Out of hopelessness is born fear. Fear that we are not in control. Fear of making major changes. Fear that we might suffer needlessly until we die. Fear of death itself.

I know what you may be feeling. Your health problems make you feel like you're in the dark, in a plane that's lost its engines, and you're plummeting toward the ground. A fire breaks out. People are screaming, and you're screaming, and the pilots up front seem to have given up. The 77 Skillful Questions are like the lighted arrows that show you the way up the aisle, ultimately guiding you to the exit doors. By illuminating the underlying nature of health and reminding you of your own deeper purpose, they even show you how to fly the plane yourself. They give you all you need to know to bring her in safely. Having clear instructions helps you eliminate the fear that limits you. If you believe, truly, that you can get better, and you understand the path to get better, you *will* get better.

Fear persists in large part because of the absence of good (and wise) leadership—instead, we rely on "solutions" that address only the short term. If you're obese, for example, and have suffered a chain of health consequences related to obesity, you might get somewhat better by tackling the obvious behavioral changes your conventional medical professionals have suggested, including decreasing caloric intake and increasing activity. I'm offering the same advice! But clearly there is more to it— otherwise you and many millions of our fellow Americans would have succeeded long ago. That's why it's important to ask the most skillful questions that go as far as possible beyond conventional medicine.

Let's go back to an early question: Do you understand the causes of your chronic condition? As you think about this again, you are probably beginning to understand that the conventional approach barely scratches the surface, actually serving to lull us to sleep rather than waking us up into a real awareness of why we do what we do and how it hurts our health.

Exploring the questions will help heal any number of areas in your life, so you'll feel less fear about your present circumstances and the future, even as you begin to get a better handle on your physical condition. When you feel you're gaining more control of your life, you'll very likely begin to take more responsibility for your health choices.

The point is, you've been on the wrong street looking for *treatments*. First, as we discussed in chapter 1, the street you need to be on is the one heading to your purpose, your special role in this life. Once on that path, you'll find things like overeating and underactivity less tolerable. In other words, clarity is both the antidote to fear and the beginning of a treatment plan for the physical condition. Once this light goes on, the way out of the crashing plane becomes easier to navigate. You feel less fear. So, yes, it might be uncomfortable at first to face your fears, but, ultimately, you must do so in order to conquer them.

Even if you're dealing with a seemingly more dire problem, say an inoperable brain tumor, the questions and self-reflection will help you, too, by alleviating fear in a similar way. By working on all aspects of your overall (mind, body, spirit) health, you'll experience less anxiety. You'll improve many facets of your life, especially your relationships and your emotional state. Nothing could be better for the body, even in the face of something as aggressive as late-stage cancer. Your sense of control and other factors of well-being will rise exponentially. The quality of your life—even if it is to be foreshortened by disease—will improve dramatically, in part because you won't be so afraid.

A main reason fear creeps into our consciousness when we begin to ask questions about our health is that on a fundamental level, we know that some, if not most, of our suffering is caused by our choices and attitudes. We feel bad about ourselves, full of guilt and shame, wandering aimlessly, living sloppy, unskillful lives. Many of our choices are setting us up for a big fall. We know we're not living our lives in a way that's very grounded or stable; we sense that our relationships are messy; we hate our jobs; we don't feel appreciated by our families; we haven't fulfilled our dreams and wishes; we don't feel connected with nature or a grand plan; so we naturally worry—we panic—that we're going to run out of time before we get our houses in order.

Another reason we live in such fear is that we're overwhelmed with information and thus overwhelmed with *choices*. Indeed, we live in an unprecedented age of information, which is awe-inspiring in many ways. We Americans collectively consume 1.3 *trillion* hours of information annually, an average of twelve hours per day per person from newspapers, TV, books, the Internet, video games, and so on. Our total consumption is the equivalent of 3.6 zettabytes per day. How much is a zettabyte? It's 10^{21} bytes, a million million gigabytes, or the equivalent of about 10,845 *trillion* words. The average person consumes 34 gigabytes of information *per day* (that's longer than this book), 365 days a year. From 1980 to 2008, information consumption grew by 72 percent.[23] In one recent year alone, it grew four times. God knows what we're up to today. And by the way, this does *not* include all the information we consume at work!

All this information is bound to inspire a lot of fear. Our hyper-awareness of every impending peril causes great anxiety in all but the most "Zen" of us. We know enough to worry too much, and this includes all we know or think we know about our health. The media doesn't help, of course, with every teaser for the evening news going something like this: "Can disposable diapers cause cancer? Tune in at eleven." We crave this kind of stuff. A few years back, there was a bestselling book called *Everything Is Bad for You: An A–Z Guide to What You Never Knew Could Kill You,* and it included things from sneakers to holy water to rain.[24] It can seem as though the entire universe is conspiring to do you in—but in fact, when you live in harmony with nature and universal laws, the very opposite is true. We're addicted to information but bereft of wisdom. It's this wiser perspective that's been lost in the sea of digits and words and images galore—and it's something we must recover if we are to have any hope of achieving the clear state of mind that will help us overcome our inordinate tendency to be afraid.

When it comes to fear, I want to leave you with an important realization. If your thinking about health often focuses on annoying symptoms; if it takes the form of, "Oh my God, I have to get this thing removed/excised/ablated/irradiated/'cured,'" then you're going to have to accept living in fear much of the time. When you begin to understand what truly constitutes your health, you realize there are many things you can *do*—and many other ways you can *think*—that will maximize both your sense of wellness and your actual physical health. You can work on improving the quality of your relationships (your spouse, kids, parents, friends, workmates, and community). You can concentrate on contributing to society as much as possible (by volunteering, tutoring, rescuing animals, just being nice to people, and so on). When you do these kinds of proactive things to improve the general quality of your life and the lives of others, your sense of purpose—not to mention your sense of control—gets a workout, and your fear will subside. What blooms in its place is a strong sense of assurance that many people would call well-being, and what I define as extraordinary health.

So, even though you've heard much of this before, it's time for you to act to gain clarity, then act on the clarity you gain.

32. Do You Have Faith in a God, Spirit Guides, Angels, or Some Other Power Beyond Yourself?

33. Do You Actively Commit Time to Your Spiritual Life?

DO YOU HAVE TO HAVE FAITH?

This brings us to the subject of faith, not the preacher's version, but your own sense of goodness in the world and in this life. Surely you have it, otherwise you wouldn't be reading a self-help book. But, this is once again a charged subject. Even if you're skeptical, please read on, on the off chance you might be surprised.

Indeed, if you want to get healthier, I would strongly urge you to consider delving more deeply into the spiritual realms. It might be no more involved than considering nature and its wonder, or a practice of gratitude. But it's worth it for the following reason: Wouldn't this life be easier if you were not alone?

Perhaps our discussion of leaving the herd has left you in a little bit of a predicament. Who's walking the path with you? Can you count on your best friends, your family, your spouse? Perhaps so, but maybe not entirely. The truth is, it's worrisome to feel alone. I think we each need to restore some appreciation for God and maintain a faith in something beyond ourselves, or we're destined for depression and ill health. If we feel loved and supported, connected to something greater than ourselves, it's easier to make real change, to commit in a real way.

If it fits into your belief system, your commitment and faith might fall toward God or your house of worship. Although statistics show recent increases in atheism,[25] a vast majority of Americans still believe in God, a majority of us pray daily, and nearly half of us attend a religious service weekly.[26] And here's where it gets interesting, from a health perspective. It turns out that people whose lifestyle incorporates their religious faith are reaping some real health benefits over people who have little or no faith.[27] In fact, a vast majority of the hundreds of studies that have looked at religious beliefs, faith, spirituality, and health, have concluded that people who believe in God or some other force greater than themselves tend to live healthier lifestyles. They are physically stronger and actually need less health care from doctors, hospitals, and drugs.[28] In other words, they're healthier.

Just how powerful do you think faith can be in self-healing? A Johns Hopkins University study concluded that people who attended religious services monthly more than halved their risk of death from chronic diseases such as heart disease, emphysema, cirrhosis, and some cancers.[29] Another study showed that frequent church attendance led to self-reporting of levels of well-being higher than those who went to church less: more frequent attendees had fewer disabilities, fewer days sick, and fewer physical symptoms of chronic diseases.[30]

Still skeptical? Then this might really blow your mind: one famous study found that patients on a coronary care unit fared better than others when complete strangers in a different room prayed for their recovery—even though those heart patients didn't even know they were receiving prayers![31] One analysis stated, "The magnitude of the possible impact [of faith] on physical health—particularly survival—might approximate that of abstaining from cigarette smoking, adding seven to fourteen years to life."[32]

Some religions include as part of their practice a focus on health. Buddhism, for example, urges adherents to purify the mind, extinguish desires, and practice healthy (essentially vegetarian) eating, all of which can benefit one's health. Several studies of Buddhist practitioners support this notion.[33] Seventh-Day Adventists are famously healthy, mainly because of that sect's emphasis on healthful eating—

also mostly vegetarian, and often vegan. Similarly, Christians, according to one study in Singapore, "[regard] the body as the temple of God so they [value] their bodies and [follow] the prescriptions and proscriptions linked to health protection sanctioned by Christianity."[34] Some of the strict dietary laws of Judaism and Islam also make sense from a health perspective, especially if you were living thousands of years ago when they were codified.

Practicing your faith and spirituality, regardless of religion, is also an important factor in achieving extraordinary health. The Singapore study reported that mere "involvement in religious-oriented activities seems to direct . . . energies in a constructive and meaningful way, preventing [people] from being consumed by trivialities and loneliness."[35]

But it's important to note here that "faith" doesn't necessarily mean "God" in a traditional sense, and "practice" doesn't necessarily mean religion, per se. It means a powerful belief in things unseen, and more or less unproven. Maybe you have a traditional concept of God. Or, maybe you're wondering, to paraphrase the Joan Osborne song, what if God is just a slob like one of us, just another passenger on the Greyhound of life? Or perhaps you find your faith among the spirits of your ancestors. Angels. Guides. It doesn't matter. What matters is the feeling that you're not in this alone. That there are forces out there in which you can put your faith, on which you can rely, in which you can take comfort, on your journey toward change. Forces, unlike the herd, that have your best interests in mind. Forces aligned with the natural order of things.

And what matters is your regular practice. If you want to achieve extraordinary health, you should make appointments with yourself and your faith, be it meditation or Mass or a sweat lodge. Put these appointments on your calendar as you would a doctor's visit—and stick to them.

And, finally, perhaps you can develop more faith in your own intuition. Maybe those voices that tell you what feels right and wrong are coming from outside yourself after all.

It all seems so simple. Eating well. Drinking enough water. Breathing deeply. Stretching daily. Believing in something beyond yourself. All of that is entirely within the grasp of even the oldest, sickest, fattest, most out of shape person out there. And yet, if you practice the lessons of this chapter alone, you'll be radically healthier than the herd around you, with very little effort and no expense. That's amazing. But even more important, you'll have set the groundwork for deep and vital change that will lead the way to extraordinary health. You'll be walking around those holes you've previously fallen into. You might even be walking on another street entirely!

PRACTICAL PRESCRIPTION 4:
TAKING A BREATHER AWAY FROM THE MOB

Picture gazelles again on the Serengeti plain, grazing on grasses and looking, to the casual observer, more or less at ease. Suddenly, all their heads pop up, their ears prick, they stand for a millisecond, inclined and at the ready, with the muscles of their thighs twitching and an eye toward the nearest escape. Before you can blink, they're all off, seemingly as one solid unit, dodging whatever snake or cheetah one of them noticed. An observer would be very hard pressed to identify, even with a slow-motion camera replay, exactly *which* gazelle kicked off the panic and set the whole herd on a beeline for the escarpment. The point is, all the individuals in the herd responded to the stress with a flight instinct.

We humans are just as susceptible to receiving unconscious and often instantaneous transmissions of stress from our hominid herd. Are we supposed to experience a lovely inner peace after riding the El in Chicago during rush hour? Should we be cool and collected when our workplace herd is terrified of the King of the Jungle who works in the corner office? Is it reasonable to expect that we can maintain a sense of inner calm and balance when our family is close to tearing out each other's throats? You know the expression, "You could cut the tension in that room with a knife"? Stresses of the herd are palpable, and have real effects on our individual minds and bodies.

Think about what happens in your body when you're stressed and feeling uptight. Indeed, you literally tighten up. The muscles of your neck and back constrict, your limbs all get stiff. Even your face scrunches up—a common cause of headaches, jaw tension, and dental problems. And that's just the tightening that occurs near the *surface* of the body. Inside, your glands and organs send a set of powerful chemicals, such as adrenaline and cortisol, surging through your system to prepare for flight, in response to whatever pain, fear, or other stress you're encountering in your environment—or even just in your mind. In evolutionary terms, this is a critical survival mechanism. We humans, just like the gazelles, have to be ready to stop munching and flee instantly if a lion shows up. And we have to be able to sense that imminent flight of the other members of our herd, so that the individual who detects the lion isn't the only one who survives.

The problem is, as we humans have evolved, most of our lions are not the real kind with razor-sharp teeth and meaty paws anymore, but the metaphorical kind: the kind who cut us off on the highway; the kind who say mean things to our kids; the kind who undervalue our efforts at work; the kind who send shivers down our spines as we listen to the anchorman at six o'clock. But the brain and the body haven't quite adapted to this new normal yet. For them, stress and fear are stress and fear.

Once you find yourself in that heightened, aroused, ready-to-head-for-the-hills state, your rhythm and flow is interrupted. Just as the gazelles stop grazing, you must stop what you're doing, too. The stressed state veers you off the course of your activities, whether work or play. It will take you a while—sometimes a long time—to get back into a peaceful, steady state of mind, so you can accomplish your goals and feel good again. If you're like most people, this happens so often that "stress" becomes a chronic condition, creating in the body a perpetual state of unease, a permanent state of worry that a lion's about to bite off your head.

The question, then, is how to come back to a state of better balance and harmony. There are a few key ways:

1. Spend time whenever you can putting things into perspective. Your boss is not a hungry lion, as much as it feels that way sometimes. Unless you're in a few particular lines of work—such as the bomb squad—your life is not really in danger. If you think about it, even your job is probably not in danger in this very moment. An angry boss might be unpleasant, but it's not the kind of impending extinction the gazelle's got to worry about, 24/7.

2. Whenever possible, leave the immediate environment. I suggest this because in our herd we tend to foster and encourage our stresses, rather than relieving them. When you can, spend a short time alone and meditate calmly on your *reaction* to the event or person that stressed you out. Why are you so worked up? What good is it doing you? What other strategies can you employ to ease tensions, to deescalate stress rather than escalate it by relating it to others and seeking their support and approval for your pain, fear, or anxiety? A short bathroom break might be enough. If you

can't get away, shut your eyes for a moment and mentally move away from the herd to look at the scene in the bigger picture.

3. Get some physical activity. This is as healthful and appropriate a response to that feeling of being wound up than "unwinding" by sitting on a couch in front of the TV.

4. Perhaps the most readily accessible—and most effective— relief can be found in the very act of breathing. Believe it or not, by breathing a certain way, as simple as that sounds, you can reverse the ill effects of both immediate (acute) and long-term (chronic) stress states.

34. Do You Breathe Abdominally for at Least a Few Minutes a Day?

Frankly, any and all of these practices can help you manage stress now and ready yourself for real health change down the road. But nothing could be more fundamental than the breath. Ever notice a baby breathing, or a dog at rest? Perhaps you can remember a time when you, too, were lying comfortably in a carefree state, and noticed how relaxed your chest and belly were, how effortless your breath was. *That* feeling—*that's* the goal.

Contrast this to moments when you're stressed: Can you feel how tight your chest becomes? How high in your chest you're breathing? How shallowly? In fact, this kind of breathing might feel more akin to panting if you were to contrast it to that same dog you saw lying on the lawn last night, mellow and relaxed.

There's been a millennia-long debate among philosophers and, more recently, neuroscientists about which comes first—the emotion or the corresponding body state. At the end of the nineteenth century, the philosopher and psychologist William James argued that the fear (emotional state) upon, for example, seeing a bear, does *not* cause the body's reactions (physical state), such as rapid heart rate, sweaty palms, and dilated pupils. He argued instead that it's the physical feeling itself that causes the emotional state. In other words, if you see a bear, then tense up your stomach, ball your fists, squint your eyes, and run for your life—*then* you will begin to feel an emotion (fear) associated with that physical state.[36]

The lesson here is that you can control your emotional state—you can move from stress and fear to relaxation and calm—by working first on your physical state. In other words, if you calm your breath, you can calm your nerves. Athletes, firefighters, police, and soldiers have employed this technique to stay focused in the midst of very high stress, even life-or-death situations. These people report—and studies back them—that when they focus on breathing to get ready for the potentially stressful event, they perform better, with more confidence and calmness. So you can practice this in bed before you wake up, in the shower, in your car on the way to work, in the elevator, or at your desk before your big meeting.

Specifically, the object of this breathing exercise is to find a way to get out of the typical shallow breathing you do high in the chest when you're stressed—and expand more of the chest and belly. Ideally, you should do this without effort (without straining or causing yourself any further stress). Many call this technique "abdominal breathing." It's the most skillful way of breathing, because it works the deep connection between your physical and emotional states. As you tune out the herd, you tap back into your life. Indeed, once you get the hang of it, for these moments at least, you are living skillfully.

So how do you do it? The key is to slow down and be as still as possible. First, take one or two intentional deep breaths, focusing on your exhaling as much as your inhaling. And with each subsequent breath, try to gently extend the length of the exhalation. Eventually, work on releasing the *effort* it's taking to breathe and see if you can just get into a new groove, gently but deeply breathing in and out. To do this, some people focus on a slow, rhythmic song in their head, or they listen to something like the wind or waves around them. You can also try a portable audio device with some gentle music or natural sounds. Once you get good at this, you can do it in the middle of a crowded and noisy subway car, just by focusing on nothing but the gentle breath. If you actually think about the breath—how it feels, how it sounds, how long it takes—your mind will quiet itself of other stresses. If you find your mind wandering or ramping up stress, don't beat yourself up. Just refocus by concentrating on the next breath again.

The next step is to get your whole body involved. Take a little survey of your arms, legs, shoulders, neck, and back. Notice any tension in those areas, and with each exhalation, relax each of these areas, one at a time, staying in your groove. Some people like to picture warm water or blue light bathing each area—use whatever technique works for you. The key is to release the tension by first becoming aware of it, then tying the relaxation to your breath.

One place we hold a particularly large amount of tension is our abdomen—so pay attention to it. We're trained to "suck it in." We're always pulling in our stomachs, and as a result, breathing high in our chests. Again, think of that unselfconscious baby or puppy—they breathe from their bellies and chests, and they benefit greatly from it.

Finally, you can add a mental component to the exercise. In the relaxed, deep-breathing state, your subconscious mind is very open to suggestion. In all cases, this suggestion should be *positive*. So, you can visualize success, and try to use your other senses, too. Focus on your purpose, and try to avoid thinking about achievement or *things*. Instead, visualize living in harmony with the world around you; see yourself as an important contributor to a more beautiful and peaceful planet; see yourself living with extraordinary health.

In less than two minutes, you should be back to center and ready to go. Try to maintain your clarity. If you have more time, use it. A half-hour of breathing practice daily will dramatically change your life and health. You can do this anytime, especially in the middle of the day when you need to relax and recharge. But if you adopt a standard daily breathing practice, such as first thing in the morning or right before bed, you may find that your stressful "blowups" become less frequent and less disturbing—clearly a sign that you're moving in the right direction.

So, why not get started? Try it now.

QUESTIONS FOR FURTHER REFLECTION

35. Are You Free from Anger Toward God?

36. Is the Home You Live in Harmonious?

Obstacles. We can find them wherever we look. Indeed, there's so much out there to interrupt and obstruct our "path" and "flow," and this causes great frustration. But what if we can find amusement in the challenge, wonderment in all that happens, as the majesty and mystery of life unfolds beneath our feet? While this might not be so easy to do on the spot, Skillful Living is defined by the relaxing of our tight hold on expectations and timelines. Let them go, let life flow.

5

REGAINING YOUR ENERGY:
GETTING IN THE FLOW

*Everything is determined, the beginning as well as the end, by
forces over which we have no control. It is determined for the
insect as well as for the star. Human beings, vegetables, or
cosmic dust, we all dance to a mysterious tune, intoned in the
distance by an invisible piper.*

—Albert Einstein[1]

NOW THAT WE'VE WEATHERED THE STORMS of denial and fear,
I want to start addressing some of the particular questions that can
help us tackle some deeper emotional and psychological issues that
tend to drain the energy we need to continue our health quest. In
order to be more successful this time than you have been in the past,
it's essential that you make sure you have enough energy to climb
this mountain. No question, it will take work. So, in addition to
the organization and coherence of a solid, skillful plan, you'll need a
significant amount of energy.

Thus, assessing how much energy you have—and where you can

recapture some of what you've lost—is critical. There are two sides to the energy equation: gaining more and losing less. To help you gain more, in this and the next chapter, I'll help you align your efforts to tap into the forces of nature that surround you. And to help you lose less, I'll outline how we can more skillfully deal with regret and resentment, the consequences of holding on to past "mistakes," and our anger—the main forces that literally suck the life force right out of us.

Along the way, we're also going to discuss the dualistic ideas of perfection and imperfection, right and wrong, success and failure, and so on, so that we can see how this polarized way of thinking can further paralyze us and prevent growth and extraordinary health. Once again using nature as a model, I'd like to guide you into a more healthy perspective, one from which we can see each obstacle or "mistake" as an opportunity for growth, and thus release unhealthy attitudes.

37. Do You Have an Awareness of Life Energy or Chi?

CYCLES OF LIFE

The energy you need to tackle life begins with getting into alignment with nature, as we've discussed. You'll experience a sense of peace, harmony, and wholeness once you begin that process. Your intuition probably tells you that on many levels, it would feel good to return to a more natural-rhythm-centered state, waking and sleeping with the sun and moon, eating naturally and in season, and spending time outdoors in natural light.

You know by now that I'm particularly interested in what happens when we adjust our unskillful behaviors more into line with nature's various cycles, which operate in a perfect rhythm over fixed periods of time—not at all like us in the modern world. Think about cycles as *the imposition of rhythm over time*. As an example, when things are working ideally, we sleep at night and wake up in the morning. What happens in our bodies during this time has a correspondence in nature (roughly approximate to the moonrise to sunrise period).

There's a long tradition of studying nature's rhythms to optimize our health and happiness. Just for example, the Taoists divide the 365-day (*circannual*) cycle of a year into twenty-four solar periods of roughly fifteen days' duration, each considered a mini-season. Internally, because the Taoists believe in interconnectedness, these periods correspond to the spine's twenty-four individual vertebrae. Taoism's two basic polarities of yin and yang balance and complement each other in cycles. Cyclical growth, one of the Taoist principles of nature, addresses all kinds of give-and-take rhythms of the universe. The moon replaces the sun, and then the sun replaces the moon. Light replaces dark, then dark replaces light. The tide comes in, the tide goes out. Arteries take blood away from the heart, and veins bring it back. These basic cycles exist everywhere in nature—it would take a library to catalog them.

From the Taoist viewpoint, the seemingly polar opposites of yin and yang (light and dark, giving and taking, night and day, man and woman, life and death, and so on) are not separate or conflicting but interdependent and complementary. In fact, one creates the other, and a little piece of each exists within the other, the way the yin/yang symbol shows us.

Similarly, in Ayurveda, the traditional Hindu science of health and medicine, we see three cycles (*kapha, pitta,* and *vata*). The Ayurvedists break the day into three segments. Like Taoism, Ayurveda aims to integrate and balance the body, mind, and spirit, thereby preventing imbalance (illness) and promoting health (wellness). In Ayurvedic, Native American, and Chinese philosophies, people, their health, and the universe are interrelated on all levels. Health problems result when our *relationships* with the universe and its rhythms are out of balance, or when we attempt to circumvent natural processes.

Underlying all these philosophies is the basic belief in an invisible, elemental energy force that the Hindus call *prana*, the Chinese call chi, the Christians call God, and the Native Americans call the spirit world. There's a basis for this belief in the most modern science: all living and nonliving things are made of vibrating atoms, and we're all connected in this way, through energy. Keeping that energy flowing, and in alignment with nature, is the basis for extraordinary health in many ancient traditions.

I don't bring up these philosophies, as valuable as I believe they are, with a mind to convert you. The idea behind Skillful Living is not necessarily to transport these systems to our culture, but rather to apply their theories of rhythms, cycles, and unity to our disjointed lives, to improve our way of life and our individual and collective health.

38. Do You Have More Than Enough Energy to Deal with Your Daily Responsibilities?

Nature never stands still. Night becomes day and day becomes night; tides ebb and flow; flowers bloom and wither; yin becomes yang and yang melds into yin. Inside you, your blood is always circulating; your body is constantly regenerating cells within its own organs; and the skeletal system is exchanging and remodeling its minerals. There's still flow even after your physical body dies.

Meanwhile, nature wastes nothing. A water buffalo is born, matures, and dies. Death might have come naturally from age, or naturally at the fangs and claws of a leopard. Once the predator has eaten its share, scavengers feed on the remains. What's left provides a feast for flies and other insects, then microorganisms like bacteria and fungi assimilate the rest. All things that were once alive eventually become part of the earth again. When the great white oak in my backyard drops its leaves in the fall, the soil welcomes this annual feeding by breaking down the leaves for the tree's own nourishment. There's a flow.

And this concept of flow is just another way of thinking about energy. Beyond this common appreciation of the flow of events in the physical world, scientists now accept as fact that space and time are intertwined, and that matter itself is inseparable from an ever-present energy field connected to the past, future, and other dimensions. This is the sole reality underlying and binding all things. And physicists now believe that the universe is connected in ways that we have yet to incorporate into our understanding of personal health. And while it's more conventional and convenient to leave this discussion out of the conversations we have about health, it doesn't mean that's the wisest, most skillful way to leave it. For now, all I want to suggest is that there's a vast pool of energy that you can tap into if you wish to. Conversely, keeping closed to the possibility, while not wrong per se, is potentially limiting. Remember the basic tenets of systems theory in question 16, which emphasizes the interconnectedness of the parts with the whole of the bike? Well, that same theory can help us appreciate the unity of all life and matter. We and all the stuff around us are part of the same great energy field.

Rabbinical Jews developed a concept called *tikkun olam,* which roughly translates as "healing the world." Today, this ancient kabbalistic concept finds its way into the prayers of observant Jews no less than three times a day. The argument goes like this: we are responsible for remaking the world whole, putting the broken pieces of the world back together into something cohesive, the way our creator intended it. The kabbalah teaches us to think of the world as a fire to which we all contribute a spark, in order for the flames to keep burning.

From a health perspective, this means that if we are hurting (not whole), then the whole world is hurting and not whole either. To heal ourselves, we must heal the world, and vice versa. This is very similar to Hindu, Buddhist, Christian, and Jainist philosophies, and that's no coincidence. Let me give you some examples.

IT'S ALL CONNECTED

As you can see, the recognition of the interconnectedness and interdependence of all things dates back to mankind's earliest and best-known spiritual traditions—and it persists in our major religions today. The ancient Buddhist text called the Avatamsaka Sutra proposes, "All is one . . . every being in the universe depends on every other thing and every other being for their existence." This sutra also illustrates the timelessness of past, present, and future as "infinite time and endless space . . . each containing each other and depend on one another for existence and are not separable."[2] Closer to Western tradition, Abraham in the Old Testament defined belief in a single God as *the* unity underlying the entire natural world. Farther east, Sufism, a mystic tradition that originated in the teaching of the prophet Muhammad, builds a foundation around the idea of knowing that all things in the world operate *as one*—and we are part and parcel of that one great energy field. Chief Seattle, leader of the Suquamish and Duwamish Native American tribes in the mid-nineteenth century, preached, "Humankind has not woven the web of life. We are but one thread within it. Whatever we do to the web, we do to ourselves. All things are bound together."[3] The Reverend Martin Luther King Jr. used this web of interconnectedness to make one of the most poignant and successful arguments ever about the state of our spiritual and cultural health:

*All this is simply to say that all life is interrelated. We are caught
in an inescapable network of mutuality; tied in a single garment of
destiny. Whatever affects one directly, affects all indirectly. Strangely
enough, I can never be what I ought to be until you are what you
ought to be. You can never be what you ought to be until I am what
I ought to be. . . . This is the interrelated structure of reality.*[4]

The idea here is not to adopt specific religious or political doc-
trines that might seem foreign to us. It's to look at the similarities in
the wisdoms that span many thousands of years and across diverse
continents, and to understand that *it's all connected*. The parts of our
body. Our bodies and our minds and spirits. Ourselves to each other.
All of us to the world around us. The world we can see and whatever
unseen world might be out there, even if we don't understand it yet.
It's all one perfect web of interconnections. When we thrum just one
thread, the whole web shakes. And when we ignore this reality, we
lose our strength. Herein lies the heart of slow medicine.

THE ZONE

You needn't be a religious zealot or even a particularly spiritual person to find amazement at some of these connections. Just think of the
human eye with all its complexity, and how it interacts inexplicably
through its rods and cones and other complex machinery with the
light of the sun and with the amazing webwork of the brain. All
around us, we can find ample evidence of these connections, the flow
of energy "in and through all things" that the Romantic poets and
quantum physicists alike have written about.

Despite some cursory appreciation for this interconnectedness,
though, many individuals still think of themselves as separate—able to
manage their lives with some kind of objective, impersonal approach,

scientific or otherwise. To live skillfully, though, one should begin to address the whole: the whole of our bodies, their interconnectedness to our minds and spirits and to the greater environment around us. Yes, this approach demands much greater awareness of details on many levels beyond the simplified, conventional way we deal with our health: "My toe hurts. Gimme a prescription to make it feel better." This holistic approach requires a willingness to do more work yourself, and to take more responsibility for yourself and the world around you. Admittedly, this could be an overwhelming project, which leads many to turn the other way. However, if we first consider the concept of flow—and particularly how we align ourselves with the flow of energy in the universe—we might find a practical and rewarding way to ease into it.

Let's start by examining the state of "effortless effort" that athletes commonly refer to as being *in the zone*. Is it possible to achieve a state of intense focus and awareness in your life, during which you block out extraneous distractions and somehow become "at one," at least for stretches of time, with some intense power? Like a great tennis player, could you find yourself in such a balanced state of flow that every part of your body is moving in perfect rhythm; each shot is dropping inside the lines; every little tennis ball appears as big and clear as a basketball; and every outside noise and potential diversion is a mere blur? Is this moving meditation, which some people refer to as being "in the flow," really possible? Can you imagine how effective you could be at your job in this state, how pleasurable this zone would make your pastimes? Can you imagine how this state would improve your relationships, your lovemaking, your self-confidence, and your health? I can.

Many people believe that such complete immersion in an experience—whether reading, studying, playing chess, singing, or dancing—reflects the *ideal* state. Can you remember a time when you've experienced this? When you were so immersed and in tune with a conversation or a project that time passed without your awareness? It's worth recollecting why and how you achieved this state, so you can get there again, get there faster, and get there more often.

But is this zone of effortless effort, which many people describe as a highlight of their life (and which religious leaders call "ecstasy"), really an ideal state? A healthy state? I don't think so. There are two significant drawbacks. The first is that it isn't sustainable over the long term as part of a healthy and balanced life, and in a sense, unrealistic. The second is that it expresses an inherent—if inadvertent—selfishness: Often it fails to take into consideration those around us. While it might *feel* like we're connected to others and the thrum of the world, in the mundane, we're really just experiencing a personal and temporary high.

Although rewarding and valuable as an experience, then, this kind of flow is not skillful to pursue as a goal in and of itself. Nearly all of us are familiar with people who get into trouble this way. After the initial thrill or high, the person needs more. They begin to seek the feeling *for the feeling*. When the admiring throngs and cheering crowds dwindle, celebrities, in particular, face a whole slew of problems that often follow such feelings. Perhaps more important, the skill or special talent that brought the celebrity the feeling—not to mention the attendant fame and adulation—eventually, inevitably, fades. What's left once the talent disappears? Even worse, what happens if the talent is lost through injury or illness, such as the football player who becomes paralyzed or the painter who loses his eyesight?

Single-minded, passionate obsession is a recipe for unhealthy living. The fiery genius that fueled Caravaggio's enigmatic and beautiful paintings, the singular focus that inspired the visionary music of Mozart, and the raw physical skills that propelled Lance Armstrong's feats of superhuman athleticism were also the vehicles that ultimately led each of these talented men down the road to personal destruction. There are thousands of others like them.

I would even debate the value of the commonly used archetype of "flow" as that of the great athlete or artist in the ultimate state of functionality. This portrayal doesn't really describe an individual living in harmony with other people or his environment over the course of his entire life.

The skillful path is not to overemphasize this kind of *flow* state, but instead to seek something more akin to *resonance*. Consider this image: It's opening night at Carnegie Hall and there are literally thousands of eyes (and ears) upon a young, brilliant musician cradling her cello. Yet she seems oblivious to the packed theater, filled with discriminating patrons and tough critics listening for the slightest mistake. Within moments, she's lost in the midst of the most wonderful Dvořák concerto. Her playing is so magnificent that the audience is drawn into a story she's telling with her cello. She's definitely in the zone. However, there's just one slight problem: very soon, it becomes apparent that her orchestral colleagues are totally off-tempo. The promise of an evening's worth of great music suddenly dissolves into cacophony.

On the other hand, a more skillful player would have sensed the problem in the orchestra, and quickly adjusted her own playing to compensate. Such a person is more in tune with her surroundings, rather than just playing solo. Such a player's experience of flow is multidimensional, and this expression of the flow state might be better described as "resonance."

Physicists describe resonance as the specific fundamental frequency created by one object in response to another (all those vibrating atoms vibrating in harmony). And as the physicists discovered, beings do not *create* resonance. Rather, it comes into play when they tap into the underlying unity, coherence, rhythm, and flow around them. We can feel resonance as a physical level of connection—as when a couple dances the tango, or when a mother cradles an infant in her arms for the first time.

The word "resonance" literally means "resound," which indicates a vibrational flow between two or more things. The commonly used expression "I feel your vibe" could also mean "I feel your resonance." "Resonance" is used in many contexts, such as in psychology, where it connotes empathy, or in the spiritual realm, where it implies a wholeness or unity of things, or a connection to a creator. Through a constant feedback loop, your body will send you physical signals when you're not resonant with your environment. Think about what it feels like to be in love—or to feel "out of tune" with your partner.

Greater awareness and amplification of this level of connection between people and between groups and other forces might help us find our way back to the knowledge and experience of our fundamental connections to one another and our environment. This, in turn, could help us make greater progress toward our common human goals, with extraordinary health at the top of the list. We could play in a symphony rather than as a bunch of soloists.

This does not mean that we shouldn't march to the beat of our own drummer sometimes. I'm not backpedaling to suggest you follow the herd all the time. But surely we can strive to be on the same wavelength as our bosses and coworkers, in sync with our spouses and children, in tune with our community's goals, and feeling the vibe of our environment. That's a healthy way of living.

Maintaining such connection to all things is ideal. This is not to say you should avoid the short-term goal of flow in individual areas such as teaching, writing, gardening, or sports—as long as you keep the *broader* context of resonance in mind. Are you really in the teaching zone if you're not connecting deeply with your students? Are you really in the flow of an Indy car race if you're ignoring what the other drivers are up to? Can you be in the flow of your gardening if it's all about you—and not nature?

39. Do You Maintain Peace of Mind and Tranquillity?

40. Can You Reevaluate Your Financial "Needs" So That You're Not Working So Hard for Things That Aren't Important?

THE WEALTH OF CONTENTMENT

When we start humming more in tune with the natural order, we can approach the kind of peace of mind that's necessary to reap the reward of extraordinary health. But how many of us do that? And how many get sidetracked in the pursuit of illusory goals like money and material goods? Despite what our culture promotes, the true essence of extraordinary health and happiness has nothing to do with extraordinary wealth—nor will even a relative lack thereof prevent you from attaining it, if you ask the right questions and strive to answer them with good sense, good science, and intuition.

Lots of studies by economists and psychologists have concluded that, assuming you have enough money to cover your basic needs, you will not grow happier as you grow more materially wealthy. In fact, I would argue that as you pursue more and more material wealth, you're likely to get out of balance, out of sync with the real valuable rhythms of the universe—and you'll wind up far less happy and healthy. Instead, you can attain a tremendous peace of mind, starting soon, if you change your *thinking* about contentment and what that would mean to you.

Taoism's sacred book, the *Tao Te Ching,* says, "He who knows contentment is rich,"[5] a phrase echoed ages later by Henry David Thoreau: "A man is rich in proportion to the number of things which he can afford to let alone."[6] This is true contentment—and lately, it's rarer than diamonds. Money is wonderful in that it allows us to afford the things we need and even want. I will admit that I enjoy my beautiful home in my beautiful town. And I will tell you transparently that I find joy in having the security to be creative and enjoy some of the material trappings I can afford. But truthfully, I understand that "trappings" are called that for a reason. I know the *less* we want and crave—the less we get used to the "stuff" around us—the happier we will be. As I write this, a few blocks away from me, in the barn on one of the loveliest (and most expensive) estates in Bedford, the police this morning cut down the hanging body of Mary Kennedy, surely one of the richest and most "successful" of my neighbors. While we really can't know all that was going on in her mind, our hearts sink at such a time. Clearly, the whole Kennedy clan with their endless stream of tragedies provides an object lesson in how prosperity, power, and success have no bearing on inner peace, balance, health, or happiness.

Today, we are so screwed up that we willingly close our eyes to life's realities in order to maintain a status quo—or to continue an "upward" striving for *more* of everything—that paradoxically leaves us far from contentment, having missed the joys of the journey. We value outer experiences and material possessions, and we routinely (and mistakenly) look to external sources for contentment. Food, cars, money, jewelry, clothing—all of the stuff that's supposed to promise us either satisfaction or an easing of discomfort. But why are we uncomfortable in the first place? We don't know, because we fail to ask ourselves.

Avoiding this trap demands that we really look in the mirror again, to seek out and then reflect on those moments of true contentment. Can you recall a time when all your yearnings were satisfied?

Remember when you were a kid, how much joy and contentment you got from your favorite toy? Remember Charlie Brown's credo that "Happiness is a warm puppy"? I know I can feel this way in my garden, and when I write, and when I become involved in helping my patients find their paths to extraordinary health. What does it for you?

While you're looking in that mirror, search back to a time when your inner world was still; when you were free from wants and cravings. Did this moment occur as you experienced the birth of your first child? Or, did it occur as you witnessed your daughter take her first steps, speak her first words, or discover the glory of a starfish she found on the beach? Were you fishing with your father on a tranquil mountain lake, or walking peacefully in the woods, away from the pressures of work and the endless pursuit of material wealth and career success?

While the elation of even the most wonderful moments fades eventually, we can appreciate that they offer us a rare glimpse of the nature of true contentment, of the inner peace and calm that is the foundation of extraordinary health. We can *never* realize contentment through external sources alone. Never. Inner stillness and peace of mind are the foundations of true contentment. "Of mind" means in the mind—not in the wallet or the driveway or in our children or our degrees or titles or other achievements.

It's important to remember how intimately this feeling of contentment is tied to our overall health—despite our specific, physical conditions. Have you ever met a person with a serious, debilitating illness who nonetheless projected a calm, peaceful, contented inner state? It happens all the time. Why? Because, paradoxically, sometimes a serious challenge to our health makes us realize that so many of our concerns, wants, and desires are petty and unnecessary.

But you don't have to get terminal cancer to experience true contentment. There are several healthier ways to cultivate it. The deepest, longest-lasting satisfaction comes when we resonate with nature and ourselves—when we tap into the source of energy around us—and when we have refocused our desires away from material goods and fleeting feelings of success that come from illusory achievements and acquisitions. *Conscious awareness*—the practice of remaining in contact with the true source of contentment—will provide the ultimate path to greater equanimity. Even in the midst of fear, misery, and chaos, we can return to this feeling if we practice it. Over time, this state of contentment becomes a new habit. The key is to give it our fullest attention when it arises. Don't you think that, whatever your physical ailments, you'd feel better if you could achieve this? Of course you would.

Cultivating greater contentment isn't so difficult that it takes a mystic to achieve it, but, like everything else worthwhile on the path to extraordinary health, it does take practice. Practice sitting quietly with nature or the one you love, or your children, or friends, or whatever "warm puppy" makes you happy. Practice simply feeling *connected* by peace and love and the simplicity of living. Practice really experiencing your senses whenever you can. Practice thinking, believing, and saying that you're grateful and thankful for what you've been given.

When you get better at this, you can try the more challenging practice of sitting quietly and continuously for longer periods. Whenever you feel yourself getting sucked into the wishes and desires that will arise, you can dismiss them, let them float by like passing clouds. True contentment is woven into the fabric of our being, and not the "almighty" dollar. Our task is to simply discover where it resides. If it suits you, you can pray during these times. You can meditate on some simple, peaceful beliefs or affirmations. Not, "I will *get* that new Mustang and that promotion," but "I am at peace."

Give yourself the time and space to practice this. The problem for us is that we're not so comfortable in such stillness. Instead, like addicts we seek constant stimulation from outside sources. Simply, we've lost sight of and appreciation for the intrinsic fullness and beauty of nature and our integral place in it. It's an interesting paradox, and a fact intrinsically tied to our overall lack of health and balance, that we tend to desire things that the universe does not *naturally* give us (a BlackBerry), while taking for granted or ignoring the great bounty that it does give us (blackberries).

GETTING UNSTUCK

A central tenet of Taoism, from which many of the principles of traditional Chinese medicine derive, is to live life in a state of being called *Wu-Wei,* or "creative quietude." *Wu-Wei,* which literally translates as "do-nothingness," doesn't imply laziness, but rather *action without strain.* In the modern idiom, it means to "go with the flow." I believe the steady flow of life energy, or chi, can open the mind and body to higher levels of creativity, action, tranquillity, and peace. Conversely, a blockage of chi can result in anger, inaction, uproar, and discord. The Chinese also believe that a stagnation of chi causes pain. Understanding these cycles and listening to our bodies' own internal rhythms, which call for adequate rest and a proper diet, can move us closer to this flow state.

If you're like most people in our culture, you're probably feeling blocked or stuck on some level. Being stuck is often a matter of habit, and therefore thoroughly ingrained in the unconscious. If we're to experience extraordinary health, we need to get ourselves unstuck. More often than not, we desire and crave things we don't have and rarely if ever *need.* So while you're sitting quietly or looking into the metaphorical mirror, ask yourself, What do I really need? Not want, but *need.* There's a very good chance that whatever it is, it's completely attainable; it's right in front of you. If you focus on that thing, you will feel less stuck physically, psychically, and spiritually.

41. Are Creative Activities a Part of Your Work or Leisure Time?

CONTRIBUTING TO THE FLOW

Now, while you're connecting with the flow, it's important to remember that you are part of the natural world around you, and nature's flow can usher out of you just as easily as it can flood into you. Finding and using outlets for creative expression, such as painting, writing, gardening, or singing, help balance us and keep us *motivated* (moving in the flow).

Creative hobbies have far-reaching benefits and can have positive impacts on mental health and overall balance in life. Creative expression is important because all work and no play makes us very dull indeed. We get out of balance if we focus single-mindedly on our jobs or other responsibilities. When we're acting creatively—even if it's at our jobs—we temporarily forget the ills and resentments and anger that sap our oomph, and tap instead into energizing waves of good feeling. We feel more confidence. We feel more gratitude. We feel more connected to the energy around us. Most important, when we're creative, we *give something back* to the universe. We contribute to the flow and the energy, rather than forever expecting it to give something to us. So what do you like to do creatively? Consider singing, dancing, scrapbooking, painting, photography, poetry, genealogy— the list is endless.

GARDENING FOR LIFE

When things are in balance, it's likely your creative outlet has something to do with your purpose, as discussed at the end of chapter 1.

In order to help you in your quest to consider both your purpose in life and options for your creative outlet, let me show you how I came to understand mine. My purpose, which I stated earlier, to join and guide others in their quest and help them achieve the health and happiness they seek, is both an inner and outer purpose. But on reflection, I suppose it's more outer than inner. It expresses more what I *do* than who I *am*. When I try to figure out who I am, I'm looking for an analogy, really, that suits my philosophy, represents my real being, and resonates across all the aspects of my life. Am I a mountain climber, always seeking the next summit to surmount? A bit. Am I a trickster, using deceit to dominate others? Quite the contrary. (It's important to ensure that your central purpose, intentions, and actions are aligned with universal morals and ethics, what Stephen Covey calls "True North principles."[7]) So am I a wanderer, perambulating from place to place in search of new people and adventures? That sounds romantic and pleasant, but it's not really me. I'll tell you what I think I am. I'm a gardener.

As I said, it's more than what I do, though I find a lot of satisfaction and contentment doing it and spending many hours each week in my garden preparing soil, sowing seeds, watering, removing weeds, and lovingly placing my plants in just the right location so they get adequate amounts of sunlight. I'm a gardener because I identify with my crops as they flourish and wither. Funny (and wonderful) that a grown man with a medical degree could find so much childlike ecstasy in seeing the first blush of pink in an August beefsteak tomato—and suffer so much heartbreak when the basil drowns in rain.

I'm a gardener because it feels like my place in the world. I like to experiment with different formulas for ensuring healthy fruition of my horticultural efforts. But I have come to accept that nature has its own inimitable design for growth—and for death. I'm a gardener because this philosophy carries over so well to my profession as a doctor. With nature's garden as a model, I have come to learn that my role as a physician should focus on working my best with nature to help my patients bloom—but not assuming I can cure every blight, stave off every bug, or control the natural designs that are far beyond my reckoning, much less my control.

I think of my relationships as a gardener might. They need to be skillfully and devotedly cultivated or allowed to run wild. Just as a gardener tends to his plot of land, planting seeds, tilling the soil, growing plants, and keeping it free of weeds, so we must tend to our relationships, nurturing those we value most, tending to those who need a little extra support and "staking," and even dispensing with those that no longer work (though I hate to think of such people as "weeds").

Now, I'm sure you'll notice all the gardening metaphors throughout this book, and you'll know when you see them that I'm busy practicing Joseph Campbell's imperative, "Follow your bliss."⁸ But this isn't about me. I want you to look in the mirror, or sit quietly and reflect on the questions: What's my purpose? Where's my bliss? Where and what would I like to create? What makes me feel most connected? What do I and only I have to give back to the universe? The more time, energy, and intention you spend on that purpose, that creative outlet, the more you will be in the flow, and the happier you will be. More fulfilled. More peaceful and contented. More energetic. And if you don't think that contentment and happiness will positively affect your state of physical health, you should think about rereading the first chapters again!

So, where does this leave you? Once again, find your passion, find your purpose, get into the flow. And then proceed.

THE "PERFECT" PLAN?

But wait. You need to be wary of one more trap. Many people are led to believe that an archetypal plan for perfect health exists out there somewhere—the "perfect" plan. Our society conditions us to expect perfection. We want things to have obvious, simple solutions, and we want those solutions to work quickly and stick permanently. Put this way, we can see the folly in our wishes. The tiny Philips-head screwdriver that sits in the bottom of my toolbox is perfect for changing the battery in my daughter's music box. However, it's completely unsuitable to screw a bolt into a steel girder on a bridge. The perfect plan, as we understand it, is a fantasy. What works for Roger will not necessarily work for Riley. And what works for Roger today might need tweaking tomorrow.

Our plans for our health are imbued with creative and dynamic forces and an energy that's difficult (or perhaps impossible) to define. This force—this energy—drives a state of constant change. And though this concept is not easily reconciled through the eyes of the reductionist Western medical model, to insist that it doesn't exist, or to suggest it doesn't matter, is not the wisest or most skillful point of view. There is no such thing as a perfect plan that can be condensed into some generic prescription. Rather, plans, like rivers, need to follow the meandering course of nature. In this case, "nature" means the individual life of the patient, taking into account all the complexity of life in general and the novelty of that individual life.

This is why my slow medicine prescription is based on questions rather than answers. This way, you can consider answers for yourself, unique to your circumstances and responsive to your intuition. Furthermore, as you change, so might your answers. Nothing in the universe is either absolute or permanent; no rules apply to every situation; and nothing can be perfectly sustained. Remember—it's in your hands, and your intuition and common sense will guide you toward the best plan *for you, for now.* It's okay to change plans along the way. It's okay to wander occasionally off the beaten path. And, as we will see, it's even okay to make mistakes along the way. It's your treasure you're seeking—and your own journey to get there.

42. Are You Okay with a Few Surprises on Your Path to Health?

NATURE NEVER FLOWS IN A STRAIGHT LINE

The thing about finding treasure is that the path to it is always at least a little ambiguous. As Gertrude Stein observed, there are no straight lines in nature. Next time you walk into the woods, take a moment to look around. You'll see that trees, flowers, and even rocks are not straight. Yet they produce amazing beauty. While not straight, they have a tendency to "flow," to work harmoniously with their surroundings. You might observe the curve of a tree branch that leads to a blossom, a smooth dip in a rock formation, the gnarled knot in a tree trunk, or the elegant dance of shoots swaying in the breeze.

You shouldn't expect a straight line in your quest for health and happiness, either. It's simply natural to find bumps in the road, curved paths, forked roads, and the occasional roadblock. Just as nature is overflowing with curves, corners, knots, and unexpected changes in direction, so our lives are, and should be, filled with unpredictable twists and turns. While you might find yourself briefly on the straight and narrow path, there's sure to be a surprise or two up ahead. Look around while you're on your trip. The lesson here is that treasure isn't always gold and shiny. Sometimes you overlook the frog and never see him for a prince, ignore the ugly duckling, never thinking her a swan.

It's also worth remembering that the journey of life doesn't always bring you closer to your goals. The hunt for treasure might cause you to backtrack or wander off in an entirely new direction—and that's a good thing. Because there's no way to predict how your journey will end, simply living is the skillful path to becoming whole—and to finding health. Like a treasure trail, this path will lead to unexpected destinations that surprise you. You might be faced with difficult questions, such as, Who am I? What's my purpose? What and whom do I value, and why? You might find answers to some of these questions after a long period of contemplation. Other answers you might discover through everyday experiences.

The path to finding health is only ever blocked when you expect a straight line or when you expect to push through obstacles head-on. Weariness, curiosity, or circumstance might cause you to alter your direction abruptly. Rather than view these as roadblocks, see them as opportunities. Eventually, everyone's journey will include a fork in the road or an eddy in the stream that will require a change in direction or a period of standing still. These are simply part of the journey. And remember, whichever way you go, there are no mistakes on this road if you know what questions to ask. In other words, don't ask, Why do these terrible things happen to me? Ask, What's the opportunity here?

43. Are You Willing to Take Risks and Make "Mistakes" in Order to Succeed?

MISTAKEN IDENTITY

Indeed, to move forward and get truly healthy, we must find a skillful way to deal with all our so-called mistakes and the unhealthy ways we feel about them. We need to question some of the ways we habitually interpret our mistakes—even calling them "mistakes" might be unskillful thinking.

"Mistake" is just a word. It becomes something negative only when we assign value to it—all the nasty baggage of our cultural interpretation. The same goes for the commonly used words "right" and "wrong." By conventionally labeling mistakes as inherently bad, as we tend to do, we actually limit our potential for growth and maturation. This can have profound effects on our physical and mental health. However, this isn't a simple matter of accepting responsibility or the consequences. I propose a complete reframing of the notion of mistakes, exposing our unhealthy and unrealistic expectations of ourselves and others. A man's errors are his portals of discovery,[9] James Joyce writes. Amen.

Like death and taxes, some mistakes are inevitable. We're certain to make many of them as we try to progress. We're rarely proud of the mistakes we make. We're usually very hard on ourselves (and on others), as we're conditioned to thinking of mistakes as a waste of time and energy.

While the typical dictionary defines "mistake" as "the lack of correlation between the intended consequences of an action and the actual consequences of that action," the definition of its synonym, "error," is more akin to "wandering" or "straying," and I would submit this is a much more skillful definition. Viewing mistakes through their Latinate origins is useful because it's in this wandering and straying that unforeseen opportunities might surface.

Some mistakes adversely hurt ourselves or others, and these certainly demand that we make amends and feel some appropriate regret so that we learn and heal relationships. However, many, if not most, of our mistakes lead us down unexpected and unplanned paths, often enriching our lives if we just open our eyes to what we find there.

I have a friend who, after heading off to college, realized that he had made a mistake in his choice of school. Yet during his first week at the "wrong" school, he met his future wife, to whom he has been married for thirty years, and with whom he had three beautiful children. Along these same lines, we have all heard about a couple's negative reaction to an unplanned pregnancy. Yet, years later, the existence of their bright and beautiful child—the product of their "mistake"—reveals how unskillful this sort of thinking can be.

One of my favorite parables, the Legend of the Cracked Pot,[10] sheds light on the often hidden value of mistakes:

> *A water bearer in India had two large pots, each hung on the end of a pole, which he carried across his neck. One of the pots had a crack in it, and while the other pot was perfect and always delivered a full portion of water, at the end of the long walk from the stream to the master's house, the cracked pot always arrived only half full.*
>
> *This went on daily, with the bearer delivering to his master's house only one and a half pots full of water.*
>
> *The perfect pot was proud of its accomplishments, feeling itself "perfect" to the end for which it was made. But the poor, cracked pot was ashamed of its own imperfection, and miserable that what it had been made to do, it could not do perfectly.*
>
> *After two years of what it perceived to be a bitter failure, the cracked pot spoke to the water bearer one day by a stream. "I must apologize to you," it said. "I'm a failure."*
>
> *"Why?" asked the bearer. "What are you ashamed of?"*
>
> *The cracked pot said, "Well, I've been able, for these past two*

*years, to deliver only half my load, because this crack in my side
causes water to leak out all the way back to your master's house.
Because of my flaws, you must suffer much work, yet you never get
full value from your efforts."*

*The water bearer felt sorry for the old cracked pot, and in his
compassion he said, "Don't fret. As we return to the master's house,
I want you to notice the beautiful flowers along the path." Indeed,
as they went up the hill, the old cracked pot took notice of the sun
warming the beautiful wildflowers on the side of the path, and this
cheered it up a bit.*

*But at the end of the trail, it still felt bad because it had leaked
out half its load, and so again it apologized to the bearer for its
failure. The bearer said to the pot, "Ah! You missed something very
important, my friend! Didn't you notice that there were flowers only
on your side of the path, but not on your 'perfect' brother's side?*

*"You see, I have always known about the crack on your side,
so I put it to good use. Every day, I dropped flower seeds on your
side of the path, and every day while we walk back from the stream,
you've watered them. For two years, I've been able to pick these
beautiful flowers to decorate my master's table. Without you being
just the way you are, he would not have this beauty to grace his
house."*

Simply and poignantly, this parable illustrates the perspective shift
that can transform the negative into a positive. I can't tell you how
many friends and patients I've encountered who've felt genuinely
grateful for what others might have perceived as a curse. *If it weren't for
cancer, I'd have never come to find my real passion in life. Without that diabetes diagnosis, I would have kept living unskillfully. If I never lost my hearing,
I would have kept taking my senses for granted.* With this idea in mind, we
no longer have to view all our slip-ups, missed opportunities, trans-

gressions, and supposed flaws and failures as "mistakes," despite our culturally preconceived definitions, biases, and habits. We are who we are, cracks and all, and each of us can find a way to water our path and grow gorgeous flowers. Ancient wisdom reminds us of the inherent interconnectedness of life, how nature doesn't make mistakes.

44. Are You Able to Adjust Beliefs and Attitudes as a Result of Learning from Painful Experiences, and Has Your Experience of Pain Enabled You to Grow Spiritually?

PRACTICAL PRESCRIPTION 5: REFRAMING MISTAKES

I would suggest that instead of ignoring, denying, or trying to wish away your past mistakes, you instead take some time to reflect on them and reconsider what they mean and where they led you. Write down what you consider to be your biggest mistakes. Put them in chronological order in a column. Then, in a second column to the right, also in chronological order, list all the things that have happened since each of these supposed mistakes—some, you might notice, will actually be *direct results* of the so-called mistakes. You will likely find a number of unexpected and unplanned consequences that resulted from straying from your "perfect," intended path, and those consequences will very often be positive, beautiful, and beneficial. Did you wind up in a new place or find a new opportunity because of something that seemed to have gone "wrong"?

This exercise helps you see that if it weren't for the twists and turns of the road, you'd never have wound up where you are right now. Indeed, all that we have today that we appreciate and cherish could have been possible only owing to all the mistakes we made on the way to where we are. So, were they really mistakes? Or important challenges and fortunate milestones on our journey? It's simply a matter of perspective.

QUESTIONS FOR FURTHER REFLECTION

45. Are You Able to Let Go of Your Attachment to Specific Outcomes and Embrace Uncertainty?

46. Do You Engage in Meditation, Contemplation, or Psychotherapy to Better Understand Your Feelings?

Return to our discussion of the medicine wheel. Natives of the North American continent envision its center point to be the site of their own heart and soul. As a practice, they imagine that they are sitting at the center of the wheel, and they recite a prayer whenever they feel disconnected or stuck in place. The prayer goes like this: "I come from the light, I embrace its energy, it fills me, and we move." Can you, too, embrace uncertainty as the light of creation, seeing the discomfort as something good trying to emerge? Can you embrace yourself and all that you feel in the same manner, and see any pain you experience as evidence of your profound sensitivity and awareness— your divine nature? Then, as a result, can you let go of the habit of self-recrimination and any feelings of unworthiness, regaining faith in your own unique qualities and qualification to be happy and healthy?

6

RECOVERING YOUR SPIRIT: DEALING WITH
THE FEAR OF DEATH AND THE PAIN OF LOSS

*I understood that within the soul from its primordial beginnings
there has been a desire for light and an irrepressible urge to rise
out of the primal darkness. The longing for light is the longing for
consciousness.*

—Carl Jung[1]

OUR DISCUSSION ABOUT RECLAIMING OUR ENERGY in order to
climb this mountain of extraordinary health leads us to the next subject: overcoming our fear of death and the pain of loss. Indeed, these
are two of the biggest potential holes that we can fall into on our path.
To be sure, these challenges are unpleasant—but they're inevitable.
We're all going to face them. So we need some directions on how to
acknowledge these potential holes without plunging into them, without getting sucked into the attendant anxiety that swirls around and
within them. Yes, the unease and the worry that surrounds loss—the
loss of jobs, loved ones, health, even life itself—is real. But it needn't
be all-consuming. The fact is, all change, including loss and ulti-

mately death, is natural. And we can find skillful ways to deal with natural change and even welcome it. Certainly change can help us learn and grow.

We all resist change and lose a lot of sleep and a lot of living as a result. We might even prefer a familiar bad situation to the promise of something better if achieving that better situation requires uncomfortable change. So, what's up with that? "Change," in our culture, is a bad word. The thought itself shakes us and threatens our vital stability. We become attached to the things we've gotten used to— even when they hurt us. And even though we fully comprehend and understand that nothing is permanent, many of us live under the pretense that exceptions can be made. For us, things won't change.

In order to overcome this unskillful belief and behavior, we must understand our *attachment to attachment.* We come into this world physically attached to our mothers, and the initial separation from our mother's womb gives us our first wrenching taste of physical and emotional discomfort. We spend the rest of our lives deeply longing to experience security, warmth, and comfort again. But too often, this deep and natural longing gets transferred in unnatural, unsustainable, and unskillful ways. We become attached to material objects, unfulfilling relationships, and unhealthy beliefs, creating the sense of endless dissatisfaction that too many of us live with—and which manifests in real and perceived bad health.

But this longing for connection obviously goes deeper than the loss of our physical bond with our mothers. We yearn to connect with the deeper source of life and consciousness that our mothers merely symbolize, a connection with which most of us in the West have lost touch, to the peril of our health. If this sounds like impractical New Age bunk to you, just think about it: Why do you pray? Why do you seek love? Why do you wonder at nature? What is at the root of your dreams, your art? What do you wish for your children? All of these uniquely human questions are the manifestations of a profound force that motivates us throughout life. We're searching for existential answers: Why are we here? Where did we come from? What's our purpose? What happens after this life is over?

These questions are primal, visceral, and inseparable from human consciousness—and much more meaningful in our pursuit of health than, say, What's my resting heart rate? But these questions are none-theless scary and disconcerting. So we try vainly to shut them up, stuffing ourselves and drowning them out with the superficial, and seek easy fixes for our immediate problems. But our avoidance of those existential quandaries has been detrimental to the health of our minds, bodies, and spirits. We need only remind ourselves that it's *natural* to yearn for a connection to something larger and more mean-ingful than ourselves. And the answers are not supposed to be easy. In fact, in many ways, the questions matter more than the answers. Finally, we need to satisfy our longing for connection and attachment in more sensible, skillful, and healthful ways.

You already know that no number of expensive creature comforts will bring back that feeling of connectedness you once knew in the womb of your mother. No "toys" or intense adventures will ever make up for the loss you experienced when you were wrenched from her loving arms to grow up and move on.

On one level, the comfort and pleasure we derive from mate-rial and sensory stimuli might momentarily re-create the security we experienced at the start of life. The problem is that to sustain and maintain this feeling, we would need to buy, experience, or feel something exciting every moment of every day. Many of us fall into the trap of seeking in vain just such a life. But without more mean-ingful, substantive, and sustainable connections, we'll go through our lives in a constant state of withdrawal, like addicts scrambling from fix to fix. That's the very definition of poor health and lack of balance.

In fact, the more unnatural and unsustainable the frills to which you become attached, the harder it will be to reconnect with the real source of health, comfort, and ease. To find evidence of this paradox, just study a young child one afternoon. Is she happiest dressed up in the latest Abercrombie & Fitch outfit, or naked in the tub? Would she rather play with an expensive electronic toy from Brookstone, or make mud pies in the yard? It's only as the child grows disconnected from such natural pleasure and contentment, and suffers the materialistic acculturation of our society, that she begins this process of transference—looking in all the wrong places for that which is right in front of her, and even *within* her. And they call that maturation?

So what will make us whole again? What will provide us that sense of security we've been missing since birth? Money and material things won't do it, and neither will rank and position. We mistakenly become attached to our jobs, our titles, our place in the hierarchy, and constantly clamber for a sense of belonging, a comfortable womb that feeds us and connects us to the pulse of the world. But we sacrifice real connection, real comfort, in this endless pursuit. We lose touch with nature. We forget the rhythms and the cycles of the universe. We trample over each other and the natural world. We don't appreciate what we have. And, paradoxically, we never arrive at this mythical place. As soon as we "get somewhere," we're overcome with the urge to move on, to get somewhere "better." Forever unsettled, our bodies pay the price: stress headaches, intestinal distress, back pain, eyestrain, inflammation of all sorts, eating away at us like a cancer.

In the most extreme paradox of attachment, we can find ourselves attached to things that are physically bad for us, like alcohol and junk food, as much as or more than things that are good, like love, community, and nature. We can even become attached to pain or sickness itself if it's become familiar and comfortable. We "cling to that which [has] robbed [us], as people will," William Faulkner writes.[2]

What's robbed us? Our parents, sometimes. Abusive relationships. Anger. Resentment. Hate. Fear. As you attempt this journey toward extraordinary health, you might already realize you've been clinging to things like these.

To be clear, it's only when we *cling* to what has "robbed us" that we get into trouble. We should strive to understand—rather than judge—our own experience of attachment, and begin to discriminate between the kind of attachment that needs to be cultivated and the kind that we need to learn to transcend. As a physician I have had the privilege of being with many people right before their death. And they get it then, for sure. So why do we wait?

MY MAJOR TRANSITION

When it comes to overcoming the fear of change, I'm not preaching from on high here. I've been working on learning these lessons myself for many years. Like most of you, I've made many difficult transitions in my life. At the height of my medical career, I was the medical director at a reputable hospital and enjoyed a successful internal medicine practice in the community where I lived. I felt secure and relatively happy in the professional, personal, and financial cocoon I had spun for myself. I had become attached to my way of life, my title, my salary, my two-and-a-half-car garage. I had reached the pinnacle of a career in medicine and achieved a level of respect in my community that others envied.

Yet behind the veneer of success was a gnawing feeling of discontent, which led me off the path of conventional medicine and in an entirely new direction—the one that ultimately led to this book. Looking back, I realize that there was a series of transitions that led me to this place. The process actually began years earlier, when I started working as the assistant director of the department of medicine at a prestigious New York City hospital. Having just completed my own residency program, I saw an opportunity to make changes that I believed would benefit up-and-coming physicians. However, I needed help with this objective from my colleagues in the department of medicine. Much to my dismay, though, many of the department's senior physicians had grown complacent with the status quo and resisted my efforts, which they interpreted as a threat to their status and methodology. They made it difficult for me to stay, so I moved on.

I left New York City for the suburban life in a smaller town. I opened my own practice. But I hit another wall, this one called managed care. During one unpleasant period in the 1990s, when the insurance companies' interference with medical decision making actually intensified to life-threatening proportions—it seemed that every recommendation I made was second-guessed by some remote automaton in an office thousands of miles away—I was dying a slow death. Patients came seeking more information, more tests, more specialists, but too often, as a result of the growing bureaucracy as well as the limits and limitations of the current Western medical system, that process brought them and me only more frustration, and very little healing. It was as though we were all running on one of those hamster wheels. It was time to change or suffer the consequences.

It took its toll on me. Even my body seemed to be telling me to stop that rat race and get off the wheel. As I struggled to employ the lessons learned during my medical training, I also struggled with a growing pain in my stomach and rising blood pressure.

This kind of thing happens to so many doctors, it's no wonder that physicians have the highest suicide rate of any profession. We're supposed to be all about healing, yet we're twice as likely to commit suicide than those in the general population.[3] Between three hundred and four hundred of my doctor colleagues commit suicide every year in the United States—roughly one every day.[4] Clearly, that was not an option for me, but I could empathize with those who gave up in various ways. My story, however, came to a crossroads after one particularly agonizing weekend spent worrying about a woman who didn't receive the requisite insurance company permission for an MRI of her brain, which we needed to rule out a life-threatening condition (we couldn't reach a live person late on a Friday afternoon). It was the final straw for me. After much thought, I made the decision to terminate my agreements with all the managed care companies and their draconian rules. I quit.

This decision led to a significant transition in my life, and put many things I had grown accustomed to at risk. I had no idea what lay ahead, or what path my career would take.

Nevertheless, I willingly gave up years of training and professional experience in favor of an approach that did not often call upon that knowledge base. Friends and colleagues joked that I was either very brave or very foolish. Looking back, I now realize that the decision to abandon much of what I had achieved to fulfill a deeper, more personal longing was not simply a choice. I *needed* to do it. Interestingly, my "ulcer" symptoms immediately resolved themselves, and my blood pressure returned to normal.

Bolstered, I wrote a letter to my patients, informing them of my decision, stating that I needed to practice my principles, even at the expense of the popularity (not to mention financial success) of my medical practice. Many of my patients wrote letters back applauding my courage and integrity. Among my medical colleagues, I became a topic of discussion. Some expressed respect for my decision and wishes that they could do the same. Some scoffed openly. Sadly, many of the same patients who had applauded my move could no longer afford to see me. Still, I felt at peace with my decision and proud of the care I was now providing.

It didn't take long before my new career hit the fast track. A new door opened, and at just thirty-six, I accepted the position of medical director at Northern Westchester Hospital, a well-regarded community hospital located forty miles north of New York City. The hospital was committed to improving the quality of patient care. I thought this would give me a good chance to influence the system from within. While I was satisfied to some degree with this new position on the institutional level, I was still troubled by my inability to answer one question that my patients nearly always asked whenever I prescribed a medication or suggested a procedure, or even worse, when I told them there was nothing I could do: "Isn't there another way?" As a career internist working within the boundaries set by the Western medical paradigm, I met so many people like you—desperate for better, more complete answers and solutions.

Honestly, I didn't know the answer then, though I suspected there was one out there. I just wasn't educated about any unconventional approaches to healing. Like most physicians, I understood that life-style choices played a role in many common conditions such as heart disease, diabetes, and cancer. However, I was still ill equipped to help people make important changes in their lives. I knew there was more to learn.

It was this growing awareness of, and dissatisfaction with, the limitations of the Western medical paradigm that started me on the road to becoming a different kind of doctor. I began to appreciate the idea of integrative medicine and soon was presented with an opportunity to study with a pioneer in the field, Dr. Andrew Weil. Weil was a bestselling author (*Spontaneous Healing* and *8 Weeks to Optimum Health*) and the public face of the field. With Dr. Weil as mentor, I began to understand healing as a discipline, and even learned to heal myself. My thoughts became clearer, my work became more focused and effective, and I enjoyed greater balance in my life. Coincidental

(I would say "synchronistic") encounters began to lead me down a new path of greater depth and meaning. My overdeveloped logical thinking brain was met by the reemergence of a more heart-centered awareness. I actually felt more human. This is sometimes tough for doctors, who are forced to suppress their humanity to cope with constant pain and death. My connections to people grew deeper. For the first time in many years, I felt sanguine about my work.

None of this would have happened had I not looked in the mirror and done a careful inventory of where I was in life and where I wanted to be. I had to stop feeling resentful and angry about where I'd wound up and become proactive, taking responsibility for my own future. I had to slough off my attachments to my training, my title, my prestige, and the *things* that accompanied all that. I had to face the fundamental fear of change. I'm not saying it was easy—but it was necessary, according to my intuition, and a higher calling.

Two years later, once I completed Dr. Weil's Program in Integrative Medicine at the University of Arizona School of Medicine, I felt retrained and "retooled." Soon after, I guided the Northern Westchester Hospital to create its own Center for Health and Healing—an integrative medicine practice. As its new director, I was able to develop close working relationships with some of the area's most respected complementary and alternative medicine practitioners, all of whom willingly shared their different approaches to healing. On our staff we had a holistic nurse and holistic nutritionists, several acupuncturists, massage therapists, yoga instructors, hypnotherapists, an osteopath, a Reiki specialist, and a spiritual counselor. It was a great team and an exciting time during which I learned a lot.

But as I delved further into the realm of integrative medicine, I grew more and more uncomfortable with the medical office label that still implied I was the "fix-it man." Eventually, I closed my internal medicine practice to concentrate my efforts on the Center for Health and Healing. I no longer tried to "fix" people. Instead, I saw my new mission as *helping people help themselves* through slow medicine. Because I was no longer under the stranglehold of the insurance companies, I could finally spend hours with individual patients. No longer was I simply diagnosing illnesses and prescribing medicines. Now I began to focus on teaching, guiding, and healing. I was finally free to help, to genuinely make a difference in the lives of those who were suffering and frustrated—people like Karen and her mother Miriam, who were some of my first visitors at the Center for Health and Healing.

47. Are You Accepting of All Your Feelings?

KAREN'S STORY: EXPRESSING THE FEELINGS

"I don't really believe in any of this alternative crap, you know."

The young mother, Miriam, had clearly reached the end of her rope. Karen, her bright, beautiful, and energetic twelve-year-old daughter, a multisport athlete and member of a traveling soccer team, had been reduced to a veritable "cripple," she said. Things had gotten so bad that now it was no longer a matter of whether her daughter would play soccer again, but whether she would ever be able walk normally, or move around without pain. For more than two years, Karen had been experiencing intense pain in her hips and knees.

Miriam arrived in my office skeptical and frustrated. She had consulted at least half a dozen specialists, who had subjected her daughter to countless exams and diagnostic tests but offered no viable answers. There seemed to be no consensus among these physicians, not even a real understanding of the problem. Miriam had even spoken with an orthopedic surgeon, who was willing to operate—though he conceded he couldn't find anything medically wrong with Karen. (Like many surgeons, even when there is no clearly identifiable cause, he was ready to "go in there," assuming some pathology would leap out at him onto the operating table, where he would conquer and slay it, a true hero.)

Out of desperation, Miriam decided it was time to at least consider another approach. That was a good enough start for me.

Looking at her daughter, I could feel both their pain. Karen walked with a noticeable limp. She winced in agony when she sat down. This otherwise delightful and allegedly once vibrant child, with no obvious reason for developing such severe symptoms, was falling apart. Every aspect of her life was diminished by this very specific but idiopathic (mysterious) pain.

Their frantic campaign for an explanation and cure for the problem was understandable. But in this case, I didn't feel that continuing that particular search would lead us to the outcome we were seeking: a healthy girl. I was also not interested in attaching more labels to Karen's condition; my job was to help her find solutions that would lead to better health.

After I spoke with Karen at length, it was clear to me that she was out of balance. My role, then, was to come up with some suggestions about how she could restore this balance, so she could get back to a healthy state. Suspending any assumptions, I listened to her talk about her life, her anxieties, dreams, passions, hurts, fears, and aspirations. Eventually, I turned my attention to the progression of her current physical condition, helping her reconstruct a timeline. In the process, several things became obvious.

What stood out during our discussion was the volume and intensity of the emotional turmoil challenging this sensitive young girl. Aside from her obvious physical discomfort, she was also adjusting to a new school, not to mention a new teacher who, she said, was giving her a tough time (clearly an understatement). She was entering early adolescence and dealing with the vagaries that come with it. There was a lot of change in her life—and, as we know, change can be frightening and disruptive. Up until this point, her athletic ability had been a source of great pride, and a means by which she fit in with her peers. Now, she was lonely and miserable, not to mention that she wasn't getting the physical and emotional health benefits of her previous athletic lifestyle.

In the dominant medical paradigm, Karen's condition would be labeled "inflammatory." And I agree with that. But the conventional *approach* would be to prescribe anti-inflammatory medications. Indeed, Karen had been given one pill after another. Looking at her challenges through a holistic lens, however, I came up with several better suggestions.

I suggested to her the easy-to-adopt principles of the anti-inflammatory lifestyle I introduced you to in chapter 1. This was a logical step, because I'd noticed a clue in the answers to an extensive questionnaire she had completed with her mother before our appointment: she craved certain foods, particularly dairy products. More and more evidence suggests that dairy contributes greatly to inflammation. And while it's not unusual for teenagers and adults to crave certain foods, Karen's food preferences were not varied, but quite limited. This was suggestive of another imbalance that is often implicated in inflammatory conditions—the paradoxical craving of the substance that produces the pain.

And there was more. I could see this girl's stress was accumulating, and I knew she needed a way to express some of the stagnant energy that was literally becoming trapped in her body—especially as she couldn't play soccer anymore. So I talked with her about the principles of Eastern medical philosophies, to help her to understand the relationship between stagnant energy and pain. Chinese medicine theory holds that certain sickness—and especially pain—happens as a result of blockage of the meridians (pathways) that circulate chi (energy) through the body. Indeed, it's an interesting question whether the energy was trapped because Karen stopped playing soccer or vice versa. Either way, it was trapped and accumulating. And beyond this, it was also clear that her energy was further affected by her feelings about the limitations imposed by her physical discomfort. As I have learned to understand, the question is more important than the answer, because the "treatment" is the same either way: in this case, getting the energy flowing was the key to helping Karen reintegrate into a unified whole. A large part of the plan, then, beyond the anti-inflammatory dietary changes I suggested, was to help her express her feelings rather than hold on to them.

The first step toward expressing feelings is to acknowledge them, to accept them as your own, without shame or other judgment. For Karen, it was natural to feel angry and resentful toward her parents, her teachers, and other authority figures, even as she simultaneously relied on them. And it was particularly frustrating for her to deal with her limitations. We all can relate. Without such feelings, we'd never have grown up to reach a state of independence. But holding on to anger leads to resentment that swells inside us, hence the inflammation. It might hurt only in your bones, but it can seep even deeper and become more destructive, leading to more serious ailments and disease.

Similarly, it's normal to feel sadness when you lose a friend, or a way of life, such as you do when you change schools or jobs. Without sadness, we wouldn't be human. But unexpressed sadness taken to an extreme creates a depressed state, which is deeply connected to profoundly poor health, making you sluggish and more vulnerable to injury and infection.

I explained to Karen that we have two problems related to emotions. The first is that many of us don't allow ourselves to have the simple feelings that are a natural, wholesome, and healthy part of the experience of human life. The second is that some of us obsess over those same emotions, turning them over and over internally, but never letting them "out."

I told Karen I suspected two things were going on simultaneously in her body. The trapped energy seemed to be exacerbated by the underlying imbalance that promoted inflammation. The intersection of these two forces was the intense, debilitating pain running from her knee to her hip. For Karen to achieve a state of better health and balance, she would need to remove (or move) some of the trapped energy, as well as moderate her diet. Now, how do you release trapped energy? How do you express it rather than retain it? There are two ways. Once again, the physical and the *meta*physical—and both ways are powerful.

Physically, Chinese medicine holds that you can manipulate the points along the energy pathways by using techniques such as acupuncture, pressure (e.g., shiatsu or tuina), and the application of heat, electrical current, or suction, in order to get the energy moving normally again. Patients often experience dramatic relief with this approach, especially in reducing pain and increasing flexibility and general wellness. For many, simple movement is also useful, and then there are physical therapies, such as traditional PT, but also massage and other "alternative" approaches. In all of these, the healing power of the hand is paramount. Interestingly, in the gospels, Christ is often depicted as a healer using his hands in such a way.

And then there is the *metaphysical*. After my initial assessment of her life situation and her symptoms, I asked Karen a question that surprised her. Are you able to express your feelings? I could tell by her body language what the answer was. I went on: Would you be willing to consider that expressing feelings like anger and fear can make a big difference in your current and future states of health? I told her that I believe they're as important as her physical activity and her diet—in fact, they're so intimately tied up with her physical health that they can't be extricated from it. I asked her, Would you be willing to try something different? To her credit, she nodded. Then I inquired whether any of her other doctors had ever asked her those kinds of questions before. She said no. I'll bet yours haven't either.

There are proven ways to release trapped feelings (which are just forms of energy, after all), catharsis chief among them. Catharsis is a Freudian psychoanalytical technique with which we're all familiar in principle. If you've bottled up pain, anger, and fear, you have to uncork the bottle once in a while before the whole system blows. I didn't want to encourage my young patient to engage in violent outbursts toward her teacher and others, but just to get some of her emotions "flowing." So I suggested she write letters to her parents, her friends, and her troublesome teacher, with no intention of sending them, but simply to express the thoughts and feelings that she was keeping locked inside her. This sounds simple—it might even sound hokey to some—but it's a powerful tool that's been used for thousands of years, since Aristotle applied it to the effect that emotionally charged characters in plays exert on their audiences. Just imagine the cathartic effect of chasing and then kicking a soccer ball—then suddenly not being able to express energy that way anymore.

And we talked. I became a confidant for Karen, with whom she could share some of her anger, her frustration, and her fear. It sounds simple, but it's true: surprisingly often, the simple expression of these emotions releases their stranglehold and makes us feel much better. Think about weeping or laughing. These are just the physical body's releasing of emotional states. You can't control the giggles—they'll eventually show themselves in physical "symptoms." But laughing is more socially acceptable—and less embarrassing—than the expression of more painful, personal emotions such as anger or resentment.

So we tend to lock those up inside ourselves. And, unexpressed in natural ways, these powerful emotions will find other ways of coming out through the body's processes: maybe stiffening the joints, maybe tightening the blood vessels in the head, maybe balling up the stomach, maybe dividing cells into a tumor.

Karen was letting it out, and she was grateful to do so. She was more willing to write the letters than give up her beloved ice cream, milk, and cheese, but, finally, she consented to give both a try, at least for a few weeks. I was impressed by her willingness to make the effort. She was willing to change, and that's a huge step that bodes very well for her future.

After Karen followed my advice for a week, Miriam reported that her daughter's symptoms started to improve dramatically. Despite the fact that she had to endure the same teacher, and continues to live through the transitions of adolescence, today Karen is free of pain. She's returned to competitive sports, including her much-loved soccer. She's experienced only a single relapse, which occurred after she had a slice of pizza at a friend's birthday. I suspect that as she finds more and more outlets for any trapped energy, some of her sensitivity to dairy products might also improve. She will then be able to live in more balance.

To this day, I don't have a clinical label for Karen's mysterious ailment. I was never interested in finding a disease diagnosis. For Karen, I found something much more important: the slow medicine path to health. I found this through focusing on restoring balance and easing inflammation by dealing up front in a natural way with the pain of loss (her childhood) and fear of change (impending adulthood). With this approach, I continually find that things fall into place. And what was most gratifying about working with Karen was the opportunity to influence this young person not just in the short term, but over the course of her lifetime. It was also a lesson for Miriam, who, like so many people in our culture today, had become dependent on the established medical paradigm to the extent that it almost paralyzed her. In the process of finding health for her daughter, she found something for herself: a new openness, empowerment, and sense of possibility.

48. Are You Aware of and Able to Safely Express Sadness, Anger, and Fear, and Do You Have the Ability to Cry?

ANGER MANAGEMENT

While we're talking about the acknowledgment and expression of all of these feelings, I want to focus more on anger, as it's the most visible. Perhaps it's the most damaging to our health as well, affecting our liver and our cardiovascular system, among other things. Most of us have firsthand experience with the destructive force of anger, which usually leads to our own suffering and often to the suffering of those we come into contact with. Unchecked anger is like a fire that consumes everything in its path. When we're lost in anger, we literally lose our minds. In particular, prolonged anger, better understood as brooding resentment, eventually intensifies our experience of fear and anxiety as we become more self-centered, separate, and isolated.

The Buddha urged his followers to give up anger, to conquer anger with love, and to avoid speaking harshly to anyone. Admittedly, this seems to be an idealistic view. The Buddha never had to drive on the West Side Highway. For most of us, the complete elimination of anger doesn't seem possible or reasonable. I would argue it's not even the goal. Anger is an appropriate response to certain life circumstances. The key is in safely and appropriately expressing it, in the right proportion.

In this regard, Chinese medicine views anger as the motivational energy needed for creativity, movement, and growth. The inability to get angry enough to defend yourself when appropriate is just as bad as holding on to anger when you ought to let it go.

This pragmatic view of anger implies that we shouldn't bind up our feelings or try to avoid getting angry at all costs. In fact, once we block the anger impulse, our feelings get bottled up, simmer in our bodies, and eventually boil over in some health crisis. Rather, we should express this energy mindfully and constructively. As long as we're alive, we're subject to injury or hurt by the actions and words of others. We should expect this. How we react makes all the difference. What's the point in holding on to and replaying your anger at others and the world? Is it hurting them? Or you? What's really getting in the way of your success—the people you're angry with, or the anger itself?

Again, this is a good opportunity to really look in the mirror and see how your responses to or actions after being hurt (or the fear of being hurt) contribute to your overall sense of well-being. In the book *Anger,* Thich Nhat Hanh admonishes, "Recognize first that the main cause of your suffering is the seed of anger in you, and that the other person is only a second cause."[5] Acknowledging and not becoming so attached to anger is skillful; it's the first step to regaining control and bringing joy and peace to your life and to those around you.

How do you achieve this? First, survey your feelings. Ask yourself how you feel about a given situation. Meditate on it. Then, acknowledge your emotions as your own. Ask yourself why you feel the way you do. What part did you play in what made you angry? With whom or what are you really frustrated? What would it take to feel less angry? Finally, express them. Not with rage or violence, but with appropriate demonstration. If you're angry, perhaps you could talk with the person who you perceive is the cause. Tell her you're angry, and tell her why. The idea here is not to cause conflict but to alleviate it. If both sides have that as a goal, this might be all it takes to prevent immediate anger from turning into long-term, unhealthy resentment that eats away at your health. There are other ways to express your anger appropriately: creative acts such as making art, sports or other physical activities, or simply writing it down, as I suggested to Karen. But, ultimately, I believe that dealing with anger head-on is the ideal method.

49. If You Have Experienced the Loss of a Loved One, Have You Fully Grieved That Loss?

A "HEALTHY" PERSPECTIVE ON GRIEF

As powerful as anger, grief can also cripple us if we don't deal with it skillfully.

Growing up, I was fortunate enough to know Jon, two years older than I, and a friend who would become an important role model in my life. There were lots of parallels in our lives, including the fact that we both became doctors. Our families were close, and my parents and siblings, along with many others in our little community, valued him both as a friend and physician.

At the exact time I sat down to write the first draft of this chapter, some fifty miles away, in suburban Long Island, a phone call interrupted Jon's weekly golf game. It was his wife asking him if he wouldn't mind stopping on the way home to pick up a pizza for his three young daughters. As he ran across the street to the pizza parlor, a hit-and-run driver struck and killed him. In an instant, his life and the life of his extended world—family, friends, patients, colleagues— came to a crashing halt. More than a thousand people attended his funeral, nearly all of whom were clearly overwhelmed by the enormity and suddenness of this loss.

I was crushed. And since then, I've spent a lot of time wondering, Why are we so challenged by the unexpected (particularly since we know to expect it)? Why do we have trouble coping with death? To begin, I believe we're woefully unprepared. Our culture avoids talk of death. Knowing that life can change in an instant unnerves us, making our world seem more fragile and less safe. Moreover, we fear the intangible, of which death is the most obvious example. Death is an unwelcome visitor, stripping our defenses bare.

In fact, experiencing the loss of a loved one might be the single most painful life event we face. We're left stunned, lost, and overwhelmed by pain. And while it's critical that we really feel our pain and loss when someone close to us dies, it's not at all uncommon to sink into long-term, deep depression owing to that loss—and here we enter the realm of unskillful grieving.

The American Psychiatric Association has even considered revising its definition of depression to include grief.[6] But is that necessary? Does our society need another diagnosis, or another reason to pop a pill? Jerome Wakefield, M.D., author of *The Loss of Sadness,* has fought this revision. He argues, "An estimated eight to ten million people lose a loved one every year, and something like a third to a half of them suffer depressive symptoms for up to a month afterward. The proposed change would pathologize them for behavior previously thought to be normal."[7]

Grief and feelings of loss *are* normal. Dealing with grief is quite different from overcoming it. There's a series of stages and realizations we go through once we face the loss of a loved one. Acknowledging the loss is an important first step, as many of us live in denial for a time. This is perhaps our defensive way of coping with terrible trauma. After acknowledgment comes acceptance, perhaps the most critical early stage. We doctors have to face it all the time, as we lose patients despite our best efforts. A recent study found that oncologists who denied grieving over their lost patients suffered a slew of psychological and physical health issues.[8] The study found that the taboo against doctors expressing grief can lead to "inattentiveness, impatience, irritability, emotional exhaustion, and burnout."[9] The study also found that the oncologists were less likely to visit their patients as the patients neared death. That's an awful shame. When patients do die, grief affects not only the doctors themselves but also their families.[10] Losing a spouse, family member, or close friend can have even more intense effects when we don't acknowledge the loss, when we try to soldier on as though it never happened.

We must all grieve in our own way and in our own time, but there are a few lessons I've learned that might help you. Accepting that our loved ones never really leave us is the best step to overcome the difficulty of grief. Avery Corman, author of *Kramer vs. Kramer*, recently discussed in a *New York Times* article the grief he experienced after the death of his wife. He was at first unwilling to let go of the furniture his wife had bought for their house. "Furniture" is an apt metaphor. Corman finally came to the realization that "her spirit is also within [my son], and his brother and me. And I came to accept, slowly, that these are only physical possessions. I don't really need to keep things Judy merely bought."[11]

That's instructive. Judy Corman didn't live in the sofa, but in the love that Avery and his family felt for her. Western culture has long pitted the concepts of loss and death as the antithesis of life and living. We do everything in our power to ignore and even negate their existence. We hide our vulnerability with fancy clothes, relationships, and luxurious homes and other "furnishings," but in the end we're still naked and frail. We still lose those we love the most, and they lose us.

Acknowledging the real value of loss, suffering, grief, and death adds meaning to life. How do we learn not to fear these inextricable parts of human existence, and instead embrace them and grow from the experience?

Western culture regards human life as a single period of physical existence. In this context, it is indeed tragic to have a life cut short abruptly. Conversely, cultures that view life as a continuum and look at all experiences, positive and negative, as opportunities for growth, hold an altogether different understanding of loss. As difficult as this is to say in the wake of losing a beloved friend under such tragic circumstances, I suspect that those other cultures, particularly those that ascribe to a less dualistic perspective on life, would likely view Jon's untimely passing as auspicious in some way. This is not to negate the intensity of sadness and grief. Rather, it's to change the context from calamity to opportunity, and use these moments to achieve a state of realization that forces us to wake up, look in the mirror, and take the steps needed to prepare for the moment when tragedy *will* visit our doorstep. Should I be interminably sad when the tomato plants in my garden die? Why? Did I really think they would survive the winter?

Failing to appreciate what we have when we have it is the real tragedy. No one should live with regret after the loss of a loved one. I often wonder what Jon might have done differently had he known that July day would be the last day of his life. Perhaps he wouldn't have done anything differently, as he was already living up to his potential, based on the number and nature of the eulogies I heard at his funeral. The real question for me is, what would those who cared for Jon have done differently knowing his time was coming to end? Did we say what we should have said? Did we express how we really felt? Did we appreciate him while he was alive, and did he know it? Did we fully love and give ourselves the best chance for fulfillment? Do we maintain hope for the future? If not, why not?

FINDING MEANING IN PAIN AND ILLNESS

Sometimes life sucks. You lose your job. Your spouse leaves. Your children get sick. You get sick. Maybe even someone you love dies. You live with constant pain, actual or anticipated. And when things suck, you really *feel* it. I'm not suggesting that you simply flip some switch in your head that will get you thinking, Hey, it's pretty neat that I got fired. Life doesn't work that way, nor should it. Instead I'm recommending you try to recast painful events, including serious illnesses, as Rick Foster and Greg Hicks, founders of the Brilliant Health System, suggest:

> *Recasting is not about Pollyanna thinking or making lemonade out of lemons. . . . There are some events that will always be lemons: sad, fear-inducing, or maddening. With Recasting we learn to deal with them as a natural part of life, extract their value, and then, when we are able, return to a happy life. We don't allow them to pervade our entire existence or become our identity. The exact opposite of denial, Recasting accepts the reality of any trauma or illness and constructs a context around it, leaving us in a more emotionally capable, elevated, and powerful state of mind.[12]*

Foster and Hicks have worked with the Mayo Clinic's Complementary and Integrative Health Program, as well as the NYU Medical Center. They frame the idea of "Recasting" into three critical phases, all of which I've used with my patients, too—even those close to death—to great success:

1. **Feel your feelings**. Dig deep. Get help. Talk it out. Weep. Write it down. Studies show that even the sickest patients who actively embrace and share their feelings live

twice as long as those who don't, and experience half the pain.

2. **Find meaning**. Ask what this trauma can teach you. Ask what you—your beliefs and your behaviors—had to do with the pain you're experiencing. How did this begin? Why did it begin now? How did it manifest itself? What does it mean? "Meaning" means an understanding of how all the pieces of your life—including this trauma or loss or illness—fit together.

3. **Recognize opportunities**. Ask where you can go from here. What can you do to make yourself feel better? To whom do you need to speak? What changes do you have to make? Who else can help? Where might this all lead if you handle it skillfully? Is there any blessing here?[13]

DON'T FEAR THE REAPER

When it comes to transcending our attachments, we can start with caffeine and Twinkies. And we can gradually deal with deeper attachments to unskillful feelings like resentment and anxiety. We can even learn to acknowledge and live with the pain of the loss of a loved one. But in this process, we need to work our way up to even more intense feelings and attachments. Perhaps the greatest of these is our fear of our own death.

We're obsessed with not dying, desperate to remain young forever, caught up in the frenzy to manipulate nature and recapture our lost youth. We spend years of our lives and billions of dollars to fend off the ravages of time, and in the meantime, we miss out on living. Most of us operate in a state of profound denial of our own mortality—and that's not skillful in the least. If we weren't so *afraid,* I think, we would be less prone to denial.

So I'm going to ask you to question this deepest of fears, and consider a different approach to aging and death—one that embraces and celebrates it as a natural part of the cycle of life. Ironically, in order to experience a sense of health, we must revise our attitudes toward death. We hear stories of people who transform remarkably on their deathbeds, healing old wounds and leaving this world with grace and harmony among their loved ones. It happens: I've seen it! The trick is to achieve this state while there's still plenty of time left in our life to enjoy it.

First, let's face facts. Whether in good health or bad, we are all technically deteriorating, falling apart, dying. It might be cancer or heart disease or simple "old age" that gets you. But in the end, something will kill you, and there's no way to stop it. A sense of the relentless nature of looming death tends to manifest in a fear of death, rather than a logical and more productive mind-set that accepts the inevitability of death and stacks the cards with skillful choices that maximize potential for two key goals: longevity and, maybe even more important, a high quality of life during the whole lifetime.

Denial seems to surface most often around the subject of death. We cover up the signs of mortality with hip clothes, cool cars, cosmetics, and surgery, and hide the reality of death by slathering makeup on corpses to make them appear "lifelike." As Professor John Powers observed in his book *Introduction to Tibetan Buddhism,* "We are even taught to avoid discussion of death, since this is seen as being inappropriate in polite company and overly morbid. Instead, people tend to focus on things that turn their attention from death and surround themselves with images of superficial happiness."[14] In *The Tibetan Book of Living and Dying,* Sogyal Rinpoche maintains that denial of death fosters a generalized state of anxiety that leads to reckless action and a loss of compassion: "We're demolishing, poisoning, and destroying all life-systems on the planet,"[15] even as we pretend we can all live forever.

In short, obsessively worrying about death (and living in a state of denial of death's existence) steers us away from the path to a more authentic existence—a life lived in extraordinary health.

For better or worse, we're the only animals that have been given the gift of knowing that we're going to die. This gift provides us with the opportunity to live in something other than an instinctual state. And this awareness gives us choices. Living without a specific, purposeful intention is squandering a golden opportunity. All of us can choose to live well with integrity and authenticity, or we can live recklessly, indifferently, and in denial.

So why are we so fearful of death? Are we really afraid that we're not living our lives now to the fullest? Are we afraid because we don't feel like we have any control? We feel we have no control because we're not *exercising* any control. We're not being proactive in any aspect of our lives, from our marriages to our jobs to our health. We're just moving along with the herd. So it goes without saying we're afraid.

But what if we started looking into and working on the challenges in the various spheres of our lives? Doesn't it make sense that if you're happy and content today with your family, your job, your contribution to society, your mission and purpose, your sense of a greater power in the universe, and so on, that it would be, to paraphrase the Native American concept, a better day to die than if you feel it's all out of control and meaningless? One of the secrets to the 77 Skillful Questions is that they lead us to a more fulfilling, happier life, but following where they lead you also makes each day a "good day to die." Perhaps it'll take you a while to get comfortable with that phrase, which I can understand. So for now, if you prefer, think about Skillful Living instead.

50. Do You Take Risks or Exceed Previous Limits?

CHANGING FOR GOOD

I know that the discussion of death can be uncomfortable. But the extent to which you "push" yourself versus remaining in your comfort zone is a good barometer for your present level of denial and fear, and your willingness to change for the healthier. I'm talking about both denying the reality of your circumstances and what it will lead to—and the fear of changing it. Studies show that fewer than 20 percent of a problem population (such as people who drink too much or don't control their blood sugar) are actually *ready* for action at any given time.[16] New research in overcoming bad habits and achieving health through motivation has uncovered six well-defined stages of change:

1. **You're in denial**. Everyone you know might know you have a problem like obesity or drug abuse, but somehow it seems to have escaped you. You're not ready to change your behavior because you haven't even acknowledged that anything's wrong. In this stage, no amount of prompting— even the most state-of-the-art rehabilitation therapy—will be helpful.

2. **You're thinking about it**. You've begun to acknowledge there's a problem. You recognize you don't want to be fat or suffer anymore from migraines. At this stage, you might not be ready to take specific action, but you're seeing the problem, thinking about the causes, and wondering how to solve it. This is a critical stage that you

must go through before you can effect change. Sometimes it takes a long time, and sometimes there's a moment of epiphany that foreshortens this stage.

3. **You're getting ready.** You're starting to organize your life toward making a change. You might be making definitive statements to yourself or others, such as "I'm sick of feeling lazy." Or you might be articulating a specific plan, such as "I'm going on a diet after Christmas." You might be buying books or reading about possible solutions on the Internet. During this stage, you're really working on overcoming your fear of and anxiety about change. You're beginning to ask the right questions and reflecting on the intuitive answers.

4. **You're making a change.** You're actually modifying your behavior. You stop smoking, or go on a diet, or start exercising. Very often, people jump right to this stage (and more often than not, self-help programs are designed around this stage, with no acknowledgment of the other, equally important stages). If you try to make some change cold turkey before going through the three previous changes, chances are that you're not going to succeed.

5. **You're keeping it going.** You've done well and seen results from your initial actions. But you realize that the action you took must be *maintained*. You hone your actions. You work on not relapsing. You appreciate your gains, but you don't rest on your laurels. You continue to ask deeper and more meaningful questions to keep up the benefits of the change. Ignoring this stage has been the bane of many dieters.

6. **You're done?** You've reached a stage where the actions you took have become a lifestyle, and you're confident that the original problem (smoking, overeating) is not likely to return. For some people (and some problems), this stage might never come, and they might need to work on maintenance forever. For others, this ultimate stage might happen after a solid period of maintenance.[17]

The important part about this revolutionary new thinking about change is to consider where you are in the continuum of stages for each of your problem areas. It's okay not to be ready to make certain changes. In fact, if you force yourself to, say, stop eating sweets before you're ready, it's simply not going to work. You're this far along in my book, so I take it that for at least one of your health issues, you're no longer in denial. You're contemplating the causes and effects of your behaviors and considering a new paradigm for getting better. Emotions, though—especially the fear of change—can prevent you from moving into the action stage. So focus on the questions here that get you to start moving from stage 3 toward stage 4, and through the maintenance necessary for stage 5.

Don't try to tackle too much at once. Instead, do a kind of personal health triage, identifying (using your intuition, a mirror, a close friend, and/or a doctor) one or two places to start. While it's true that action cures fear, don't act until you're *emotionally ready* to act. Don't beat yourself up if you're not quite ready. You're only human.

Having said that, don't wait until it's too late to act. Use your intuition and skillful self-questioning to reveal to you where you must act—and act relatively soon. Then try to push yourself just a little bit more each day. Maybe you're not entirely ready to act on adopting an extraordinarily healthy diet cold turkey, starting today. But we eat one meal and one snack at a time. So here, "exceeding previous

limits" means allowing yourself the responsibility to make some better choices, one at a time. So you've snatched a handful of candy from
that bowl at the bank: Does that mean you have to eat another, and
another, and then go out for a pizza?

Finally, a word on taking risks. The risks I'm talking about here
are not like BASE jumping or swimming with sharks. I'm talking
about acknowledging the fears you live with daily, and taking slow,
safe, and incremental steps to overcome them on your path to extraordinary health.

51. Do You Have the Ability to Concentrate
for Extended Periods of Time?

FOCUS AND HEALTH

It took Karen a considerable amount of time and energy to focus on
her problems, rather than denying them. And it might for you, too.
The solutions, too, as we've seen from the new research on changing
our behaviors, often take prolonged concentration, which is in short
supply these days. Who has the time to sit down and focus on one
particular task anymore, even when we know it's imperative? We live
in a multitasking age, with around-the-clock access to the world at
our fingertips, and a barrage of devices and temptations yelping for
our attention.

Multitasking is a myth. You don't need to consult a hundred studies to understand that. Just look at your cell phone (which you often
do when you should be paying attention to your work, your health,
your kid, your spouse, or your driving). We think we can do it all,
but studies show we can't very well.[18] It's not natural. Our brains have

a built-in bottleneck against multitasking. You can't exactly compose a poem for your cave-wife while you're trying to outrun a woolly mammoth. Nor can you effectively compose a text message while you're driving at sixty-five miles an hour. Trying to do more than one thing at the same time leads to a gross loss in efficiency.[19] It can cost us 2.1 hours of our day, and it costs the economy $588 billion each year.[20] But multitasking and lack of focus and concentration aren't only costing companies money—they're costing us our health and sanity. In the case of texting while driving and other extreme examples, they can cost us our lives. More subtly and more commonly, they create psychological and physical health deficits in people that we're just beginning to understand.

Just look at the number of people who exhibit the symptoms of attention-deficit disorder (ADD), often called attention-deficit/hyperactivity disorder (ADHD). Many of these patients cannot be clinically diagnosed with ADD/ADHD because they have no inherent brain or nervous system defect: The ADD/ADHD symptoms are *created* by the physical and environmental factors[21] we all face nowadays. In other words, it's the modern world that's making us this way.

In fact, recent studies show that these ADD/ADHD symptoms are more prevalent in developed countries, such as in the West.[22] L. Alan Sroufe, a psychologist, explains in a recent article in the *New York Times* that "findings in neuroscience are being used to prop up the argument for drugs to treat the hypothesized 'inborn defect.' These studies show that children who receive an ADD diagnosis have different patterns of neurotransmitters in their brains and other anomalies. . . . Of course the brains of children with behavior problems will show anomalies on brain scans."[23] But it's not as simple as a physical problem in the brain, but also the brain responding to challenges in the modern world.

It's clear to me as a physician that we have an integrated problem that requires an integrative solution. But what about our lifestyle is causing either these inborn defects or similar symptoms to develop in people with no genetic markers or history of ADD/ADHD? As Dr. Edward Hallowell points out in one study, a leading factor is anxiety,[24] which makes perfect sense to me.

Anxiety is universal to both adults and children. Anxiety about what? Our performance. Fear of what others are thinking about us. Fear of losing our jobs. Fear of being rejected by our choice of school or mate or . . . fill in the blank. In short, when we're anxious, we can't focus. When we can't focus, we can't perform. And when we can't perform, we get down on ourselves even more, losing even more ability to focus, and we wind up in a never-ending spiral.[25, 26] Very soon, the stress of this situation causes physical symptoms. Sleep disorders. Headaches. High blood pressure. Infections. Inflammation. The whole panoply of Big 8 conditions.

If you find you can't focus for sustained periods, if your concentration is weak, you're likely experiencing some anxiety, and it's worth trying to get to the bottom of that before you move on. Look in the mirror or just slow down for a moment: What are you afraid of? At first, it might seem like you're afraid of failing the "test," but if you drill down, your real fear is about death and dying. And before that, the pain that threatens loss and the anger and frustration and grief that result.

PRACTICAL PRESCRIPTION 6:
ENVISIONING EXTRAORDINARY HEALTH

This prescription uses a technique called guided imagery, a program of directed thoughts and suggestions that guide your imagination toward a relaxed, and focused state. For some reminders about how to achieve that state, you might want to review Practical Prescription 4 on page 154.

Guided imagery relies on an understanding of the mind-body connection. The mind cannot distinguish between "real" and "imagined" when you employ all your senses. In other words, if you picture something—and really see, feel, hear, and even taste it—the mind interprets this as real, and responds accordingly. You know this to be intuitively true. If you really imagine your grandmother's cooking—really remember the smell and the taste and the feel of her food in your mouth—you're liable to salivate. Similarly, if you imagine something terrible happening—a fire in your home or your child in an accident—your blood pressure goes up, your heart beats faster, and you might even start to sweat.

The idea here is to guide your imagination toward the peaceful, relaxed, and positive, of course. You can get to this state by using all your senses to imagine a safe, comfortable environment, such as a mountain lake or your childhood bedroom—whatever works for you. Start with your favorite peaceful place, then expand this vision:

Envision a world that's in greater harmony and resonance, one that supports a divine plan of creation, that includes even more beauty and wonder, in which you and all other beings get to fulfill their purpose. A world where you and others are free of fear and pain. What would this world look like, feel like, sound like?

Now envision your role there. Envision a world where you are very aware of your distinct role in supporting this plan. What are you doing in your ideal, healthy, balanced world? What do you look like? How does it feel?

Now bring an awareness into your vision, that your health is intricately connected to your relationship to others and to the greater cosmic reality. Try to feel the energy all around you. Whatever anxiety and pain you experience goes well beyond your physical symptoms, though these play an important role in your process, if only you could learn, grow, and transcend them. Envision your particular circumstance now and witness it dissolve into the light source around you. Repeat to yourself that your health is not as severely limited by age, disease, or even death as you have been taught. There is so much more to your existence. Bring to mind your purpose. Reassure yourself that there is no need to give up trying to alleviate your discomfort. But there are other questions to ask that will contribute to your healing. Don't lose sight of those, and see how, one by one, you step closer and closer to that state of harmony and resonance you seek—the feeling of security, warmth, and comfort you experienced just before birth.

This kind of guided imagery with its related relaxed state can aid healing and lead to extraordinary health. It can help with learning, with creativity, with performance, and in our efforts to change. I have found that it helps people face their challenges—even the big ones—to recover their spirit.

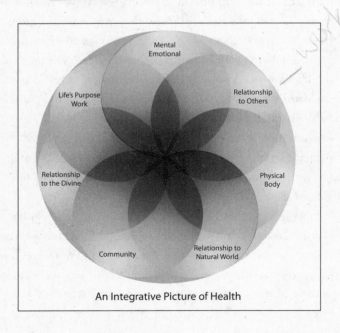

An Integrative Picture of Health

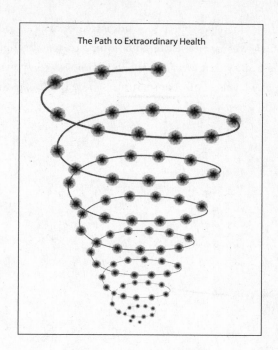

The Path to Extraordinary Health

QUESTIONS FOR FURTHER REFLECTION

52. Is Your Sleep Free from Disturbing Dreams, and Do You Explore the Symbolism and Emotional Content of Your Dreams?

53. Are You Free of Any Drug or Alcohol Dependency (Including Nicotine and Caffeine)?

Nightmares. We don't ask for them, but they happen nonetheless. Are we courageous enough to hear and heed their messages? Are we wise enough to listen without judgment and with curiosity? Similarly, can we accept ourselves when our addictive behavior leads us into darkness? Can we maintain the equanimity to see through the veil and find the beauty that awaits us when we choose to evolve? Indeed, there are many levels of our consciousness. The idea is to look at them all, learn, and grow.

7

ACCEPTING YOUR FAMILY AND CULTIVATING YOUR RELATIONSHIPS: WHERE YOU CAME FROM AND WHERE YOU ARE NOW

The quality of your life is the quality of your relationships.

—Anthony Robbins[1]

WE'VE TALKED AT LENGTH ABOUT EXPRESSING our feelings and effecting changes in order to navigate back on track to a better life for ourselves. But why are we so vulnerable to being derailed in the first place? That's a complicated question, but we can answer it in simple ways. Starting when we're young, we begin to accumulate the various slings and arrows that others shoot our way, whether deliberately or not. The people around us affect us. Their arrows can wound us and hinder our progress just as easily as their embraces can heal our pains.

So I'd like to turn our attention now more deeply to this web of relatedness in which we all exist—the web that so profoundly influences who we are and how we feel. Although we're responsible for our own health, our own feelings, and our own changes, none of these things are isolated elements, because none of us lives in isolation. As the poet John Donne writes, no man is an island. We're all part of the same "continent," intimately and intricately connected to each other and the world around us. It's true that the strength of the fibers of those connections—of our past and present relationships—are as sure a sign of our overall health as our blood sugar or body mass index.

Because relationships are fundamental to the fabric of life, their success is a great yardstick by which to measure our personal growth and health. Sound, healthy relationships require compassion, balance, flexibility, and equanimity. Indeed, not only do our relationships reflect the quality of our lives, they are the most accurate way to assess and measure our state of health.

You must remember, though, that this web of interconnectedness works both ways. Dysfunctional or absent relationships inform us that something is amiss in our personal health and growth. So I'll also be reminding you to spin out *your* silk and make filaments between you and those around you; the strengthening of these bindings ensures our health and survival. But just as much or more so, we need to consider our early bonds, too, sometimes shoring them up and sometimes severing them if they were built on foundations that were so unskillful, they can't be fixed.

Although we live in a world that values rabid individualism—and such individualism has its place in healthy development—it's a linchpin of the new and skillful health paradigm that understanding health requires that we understand our relationships. That means the family relationships that shaped where we came from, the intimate relationships that shape our present circumstances, and the community of relationships in which we would like to live. You know this to be intuitively true: it's nearly impossible to experience a state of health if our marriages are destructive, the people we work with are "psychic vampires," and our cities and social establishments are in ruin. And all this interconnectedness starts with how we grew up—our first community, our family of origin.

54. Did You or Do You Feel Close with Your Parents?

WHERE YOU CAME FROM: ACCEPTING YOUR FAMILY

The foundation of all human relationships is the relationship between parent and child. Although the following questions can sometimes cause pain, I want to encourage you to ask yourself where you came from, and consider how your primary family relationships are contributing to your physical health, happiness, and emotional well-being today. As children, our autonomy can be stunted by well-meaning but overbearing and overprotective parents. And we can be victims, form unhealthy attachments to victim mentalities, or develop other forms of chronic negativity and pessimism based on our early experiences of repression, abandonment, anger, fear, and so on.

In the worst case, we can suffer outright abuse and terror from those who were supposed to protect us. On the other hand, our parents can work miracles, helping make us self-possessed, self-actualized, whole, and healthy adults. In any case, there's no doubt our families shape us—but they needn't limit us. We *can* transcend them.

So to begin with, I want you to spend some time thinking about your relationship with your parents when you were a child. How did your parents treat you? How did you feel when you were with them? How would you assess their parenting skills? Here are some more specific angles, in black and white, from which to view your parents and the way they reared you. Your memory and intuition will help you determine where your parents fell on the continuum between these extremes:

THE SKILLFUL PARENT	THE UNSKILLFUL PARENT
Respects and recognizes the integrity and autonomy of the child from the very first moments of life, writing a recipe for future independence, health, balance, and high self-esteem.	Considers the child only as an extension of self, compelling the parent to "manage" every aspect of the child's life, often well into adulthood, "for their own good," producing a resentful, rebellious, confused person, with low self-esteem.
Prepares the child to enter the real world by allowing her to learn age-appropriate lessons, and sometimes experience necessary pain in order to grow stronger.	Infantilizes the child, shielding her constantly, overprotecting and overcontrolling, perpetuating dependency and an inability to problem-solve in later life.
Models the kind of person he wants his child to become; behaves as a role-model as much as possible in matters of integrity, honesty, good citizenship, hard work, and health, making for a child who follows suit and feels internally good about herself as she moves through life.	Never considers ethical modeling, frequently "slips" in morals, behavior, beliefs, and speech, offering repeated unskillful examples of behavior and thought that a child can mimic, stymieing her later development.
Provides stability in his relationship with his family of origin and the other parent, as well as in finances, beliefs, and in a harmonious and established home that offers the child consistency and steadiness to build on as she grows.	Creates an unstable environment with different partners, constant moving, lack of enough money, constantly wavering beliefs, and fighting with his own family, upending the child's sense of safety, stability, and harmony.
Shepherds good health in the home by making skillful choices about food, physical activity, natural healing, and medicine, ensuring skillful choices in the child's later life.	Exemplifies poor, unhealthy, and unskillful choices about diet and exercise; doesn't take responsibility for the young child's health; models Band-Aid solutions to medical challenges, setting the child up for immediate and long-term physical health challenges.
Demonstrates an ability to show love, both physical and emotional, with the other parent and with the children in the home, increasing the chances the child will form healthy, loving relationships in her future.	Withholds love in order to "toughen" the child; is physically, emotionally, or sexually abusive; acts distant for whatever reason, setting the child up for bad relationship choices and failure and pain in future relationships.

THE SKILLFUL PARENT	THE UNSKILLFUL PARENT
Disciplines the child firmly, fairly, and consistently when necessary, teaching consequences for unskillful actions, thus demonstrating love and care for the child's future, helping the child understand responsibility and the costs of poor choices.	Allows bad behavior and unsafe decisions to go unpunished, or inconsistently or unfairly punishes actions, setting up a frightening, unsafe, and out-of-control world for the child, which can lead to an undisciplined adulthood.
Expresses emotions like pain, fear, and anger regularly and in appropriate and moderate proportions; discusses these emotions and their meanings with the child, and allows the child the space and consideration to share her feelings, too, setting her up for an emotionally rich and healthy later life.	Swings wildly with emotions, or bottles them up and never expresses them; scolds the child for her expressions of emotions, and confuses her about her feelings, setting her up for future misery.
Forgives the child easily, even when the child must be disciplined, teaching valuable lessons about love, trust, and intimacy.	Holds grudges; blames the child for his own feelings, creating a resentful, shame-filled, and agonized child who will have trouble dealing with adult emotions appropriately.

Chances are, your parents fell somewhere in between the columns. However they performed, you didn't have much choice in the matter. But we can see here how the choices they made had a profound impact on the way we turned out. The good news is that we're not children anymore. We're not cowering in a corner, or silent at the table, or acting out at school. We're (more or less) fully formed adults with the ability to choose now for ourselves. We can act responsibly now, taking our lives and our actions and beliefs into our own hands. This is critical, because the past relationships with your family of origin remain very much alive and active in your chosen relationships now. To move forward in those relationships, you must first come to terms with the past.

So I'd recommend you first come to terms with the mistakes made by your parents. I'd like to be able to assume that, like most parents, they did the best they could, and occasionally made some mistakes that might have hurt you, but overall, if you're reading this, there's good reason for optimism. But I know it's not that simple. Truthfully, some parents should never be parents. I hope that your childhood was not overtly abusive and awful, but I know that it might have been. If you think about it, the very nature of childhood is "abusive" to some degree, at the very least repressive. As a young child growing up in our culture, you're essentially living entirely at the whim of the adult world, with very little say over anything in your life: even the most essential choices like where and when you sleep and eat are made by your "overlords." Whatever your childhood circumstances were—even if they were dire—you can accept that it was what it was, mistakes and all, and get yourself ready to move on. You see, it doesn't really matter what happened to you, what was done to you when you were a child, because now you're an adult, no longer actively subjected to those mistakes—unless *you* continually allow them in your life. You cannot change one iota of the past. The only thing over which you have any control now is the way you deal with your childhood. Even if you have recurring nightmares and can't easily overcome the subconscious and unconscious effects, there's more you can do to change the way the past haunts your present.

If your parents are still alive, you might consider speaking with them about your discoveries when you reflect on this question. If you have to talk to a tombstone or a photograph, you can still gain a lot from that catharsis. If it's easier and more comfortable for you to write down your feelings or discuss them with a therapist, close friend, or spouse, do that. Just don't keep it in any longer. Your body, mind, and spirit will all thank you.

As you learn lessons about how your parents handled or mis-handled you as a child, you can hone your own parenting skills, if it applies. If you yourself have made the choice to be a parent, now you're responsible for the health of your children and those around you who can't take complete care of themselves, and who will someday become adults themselves. What would you like your children to say about you at your gravesite? There's¹ much more on the subject of skillful parenting that I'll share in a future book. But for now, start here.

55. Can You Forgive Yourself and Others?

Forgiveness is the virtue of the brave.

—MAHATMA GANDHI²

In the ideal scenario, you will find a way to forgive your parents. You could consider that your parents were only human. They were as messed up and pained as most people, and, for the most part, most of them tried to do the right thing, at least most of the time. But even if they didn't—even if they were blatantly terrible to you—you can still learn to forgive. Many millions have, using their faith or meditation or professional counseling or the love of a good spouse to help. While most of us would agree that perhaps the worst thing a person can do in this life is to harm a defenseless child, we might also agree that one of the worst tragedies is that child holding on to the pain until the day he dies, an old and miserable cuss. You bring yourself your life. Now, as an adult, *you* and only you can bring yourself peace and forgiveness.

The same goes for pains you've suffered at the hands of others, besides your parents. Yes, it hurts to be wounded. But we all know that wounds must be tended—cleaned, stitched, soothed, and salved, until they scab over. You wouldn't tear off a scab daily and dig through a physical wound with sharp nails, would you? So why would you go out of your way to aggravate a psychic wound by rehashing and daily reliving the pains of the past? Yet that's exactly what you do in your head and your heart with daily reminders of how you were hurt way back when. That was yesterday. Today is today, and you should assume there will be a tomorrow.

Common sense would compel you to cast off something immediately dangerous to your life and health. If someone handed you a ball of fire, instinct and the autonomic nervous system would cause you to hurl it out of your hands before you could blink—before you could even *think*. If you swallowed some toxin, the body's defenses would force you to vomit it out of your system as soon as it was detected. Even on the cellular level, the body acts to fight microinvaders and predators, sending white blood cells on assassin missions. If any of the systems failed, we'd say you had a grave health crisis, and the system was in need of urgent aid. In this context, it's a strange paradox that when it comes to psychic and emotional dangers, we tend to hold on, rather than cast off. We keep that poison inside us, churning. We hold onto that fireball, which burns us. We let the toxin into every fiber of our being. That, too, is a sick system in need of healing.

I know it isn't easy, and it sometimes takes years—and the help of a professional—but there are few things that will contribute to your health and increase your quality of life more powerfully than forgiveness, more healing than letting go of the past. Yes, we've all been wounded in some way, sometimes severely. And, yes, we feel damaged. Somebody abused us, or took something from us. But now it's over. Now it's up to us. If we fan those flames, if we keep swallowing that venom, we're going to suffer indefinitely, and for what? Does that hurt our parents or our abusers or our ex-spouses or whoever mistreated us? Absolutely not. It only feeds the hungry monsters inside us, whom we've invited to take up residence in our souls. They eat away at our lives. They eat our time. Our energy. Our self-esteem. Our ability to love. We suffer disturbing dreams and phobias. We get depressed. We endure panic and anxiety attacks. We develop obsessive-compulsive behaviors. We overeat and engage in risky sexual behaviors.

And these monsters consume our bodies, too. They eat away at our stomach lining and feed cancers. We watch our blood pressure and our heart rate rise. To paraphrase Dante, the putrid slime from the mouths of these hungry ghosts boils and swells inside us, in the form of abscesses and infections. Indeed, those monsters made out of holding on to past pain are often at the root of our maladies, from our head down to our toes. As hard as we might try to push them away, hold our breath, or just simply bear the pain, we ultimately succumb. Perhaps it's no surprise, then, that the two most common areas at risk from this "holding on" are our lungs and colon—the organs responsible for letting go.

Think about it: What would happen if you never exhaled or released what was in your bowels? That's the experience of holding on to the mistakes of the past. We get full of gas, congested, constipated, stagnant, and toxic. So we've got to let. There's a profound relief and a massive physical and emotional benefit in forgiveness and other forms of letting go. I can't think of a pill I've ever prescribed that can have as profound an effect.

So get back in front of that mirror. Think about the past pains and hurts you're holding on to. Who's out there to forgive? Did they send you away to school when you wanted to stay home? Did they treat your sister better? Did they forbid you dating that girl you liked? Did they hit you? Molest you? Abandon you?

Maybe you need look no further than the mirror—maybe it's time you forgive *yourself* for some past mistake.

If you don't feel quite ready to forgive yet, you can recognize that you can still *let go* of those things you can't change. You must. What are the other choices? A lifetime of suffering like a helpless child, full of bile and stagnant air? If you learn to let go—with professional help, if you need it—you take responsibility for your now and your future. You take the wheel, the reins, the rudder—whatever cliché you want to use. You take back your life, and your health.

56. Do You Enjoy High Self-Esteem?

57. Do You Experience Unconditional Love?

MADE IN "USA"

Letting go of toxins, both emotional and literal, will make you feel better. An obvious factor in good health is feeling good about yourself, and vice versa. So let's talk for a moment about an often misunderstood notion called *self-esteem*. Not surprisingly, several key studies conducted on adolescent and adult behavior show that low self-esteem is a factor in the development of depression[3] and other disorders. It works the other way around, too: depression likely leads to low self-esteem, which further increases the depression, spinning out a negative spiral that can lead to suicide or a completely wasted, "frozen" life.

On the other hand, studies conducted on adolescent behavior have observed that high self-esteem increases happiness in all aspects of life.[4] How do you get it? Well, if you lead an active life, with intimate relationships with parents, friends, and romantic partners, you're going to experience higher levels of self-esteem. And such high self-esteem will in turn benefit your relationships and your quality of life, a fulcrum in extraordinary health.

It's critical that you achieve this, even if you have to get there incrementally. Low self-esteem has been linked to increased susceptibility to all kinds of illnesses of the mind and body. Michael Marmot, the previous director of the British Medical Association, cites a study of two groups of Pima Indians in Arizona who had high levels of obesity and diabetes. One group acted as the control group, while the other was provided support in maintaining a better level of health. At the end of the study, researchers concluded that "increasing pride in their identity had a more favourable impact on health behaviours and risk than focusing on how to change diet and exercise."[5] I've studied the outcomes in thousands of my own patients and seen similar results: maintaining a positive view of yourself—improving your self-esteem—leads to improved mental *and* physical health.

But what exactly is self-esteem? Is it hubris? Didn't such excessive pride kill all those Greek heroes and Shakespeare characters? Isn't it pride that goeth before the fall, turning Lucifer to Satan? Is it vanity, narcissism, conceit? How can any of that be healthy?

Albert Ellis, the famous humanist and founder of the Rational Emotive Behavioral Therapy school, answered that question. He built a sixty-year career on one simple principle that attracted millions of adherents: Unconditional Self-Acceptance, or USA. Ellis argued that happiness, balance, and health are indeed dependent upon high self-esteem, and the only way to truly attain a high sense of self-esteem is to forgive and accept yourself *unconditionally:*

> *Give up all your ideas about self-esteem, stick only to those of unconditional acceptance, and choose to accept your self, your existence, your humanity whether or not you perform well, whether or not you are loved by significant others, and whether or not you suffer from school, work, sports, or other handicaps.*[6]

In other words, don't tie how you feel about yourself with how "good" or "right" you are, because you *are* yourself, a self worthy of your own esteem. Psychologist David Mills expands on his mentor Ellis's theory by explaining that "most people unfortunately believe that self-esteem must, in some way, be *earned through achievements*."[7] You know how this works: You lose five pounds, so you feel good about yourself. But later, you eat twelve cookies, and now you feel bad. There are three fundamental problems with this very common way of thinking. The first is that it's a false dichotomy:

> *To overcome self-esteem-related anxiety and inhibition, recognize that your choice is not between self-esteem and self-condemnation. Your choice, rather, is between establishing an overall self-image and establishing no self-image. That is, you can choose to view your external actions and traits as desirable or undesirable, but abstain from esteeming or damning yourself as a whole.*[8]

Which leads to the second problem with that good/bad dichotomy: it shouldn't be the point of self-esteem in the first place. It's called "self"-esteem and not "action"- or "belief"-esteem for a reason. You need to feel good about your *self*, even if you don't feel that you've made an ideal *choice* in any given situation. In other words, you can criticize and challenge your behaviors—"Eating three croissants was not the smartest move in light of my weight-loss goal"—without criticizing or challenging your *self*—"I'm a big, fat, ugly, stupid failure."

Lastly, there's a problem with the quest itself for self-esteem. As Mills writes, "A compulsive drive for self-esteem leads to increased anxiety. And self-esteem-related anxiety is an obstacle to achieving those goals so essential to our self-esteem!"[9] So don't fret about it or overanalyze it. Just practice, daily—or several times a day until it sinks in—some USA. Speak kindly to yourself. Tell yourself you're okay. Yes, not every choice you've made so far has been skillful, but *you* are a good person, deserving of your own esteem just because you're you. If some of your choices need honing, that's all right. Start making those changes. Just remember, that's about your decisions, your behavior, your actions, which might need some changes—not your core *self*, which you should accept *unconditionally*. It's uncertain if you'll ever experience unconditional love from someone else, so you should at least get it from yourself.

58. Do You Give Yourself More Supportive Messages Than Critical Messages?

FLIPPING THE SCRIPT

If you don't accept yourself—if you don't forgive yourself and learn to like and care for yourself—then your physical body, and your mind and spirit, will never heal. They won't be able to help you, because they will have received the message loud and clear that you're not worth it.

There's a valuable slow medicine prescription I can offer here to help you on the way to USA: It's called *positive self-talk*. This is just a fancy way of saying you need to be nice to yourself. We all have continuing "scripts" in our heads, consisting of our inner self-talk. The things you say to yourself on an ongoing basis need to be supportive, loving, fair, and kind—not hateful, shame-inducing, and mean. It's that simple. Skillful Living and extraordinary health rely on a sense of self-worth that springs from the reminders you give yourself often about who you are and what you're worth. So sit down somewhere quietly, in a comfortable room or out in nature, and listen to yourself talking to yourself. What do you say to the you in the mirror? What messages do you give yourself? As you slowly become aware of these messages, work on altering them. Although they seem to work on an unconscious level, they're entirely within your control. Look at the difference between positive self-talk and negative self-talk:

SKILLFUL SELF-TALK	UNSKILLFUL SELF-TALK
I made a good choice at dinner tonight, avoiding that second glass of wine.	I'm a useless drunk and I'll never get it under control.
Cooking with all this salt is not the most skillful choice for my high blood pressure. Cutting down will help my health.	I'm addicted to salt. I'll never be able to give it up.
I'd like to be more patient with my kids. The weekend was peaceful, but come Monday, they were really pushing my buttons. I'm going to work on ways to see things more from their perspective before I yell.	I'm a terrible parent.
I've been procrastinating on getting my health in better shape. Today I'm going to start with something simple and positive, walking to lunch instead of driving.	I'm so lazy and useless—I can't even take care of my own health.

Notice how positive, skillful self-talk, even when it must be self-critical, accentuates the positive, focuses on changeable behaviors that lead to desired outcomes, and works on finding a path to solutions. It doesn't attack *you*, the person behind the decisions. Negative, unskillful self-talk, on the other hand, goes right for the jugular, savaging your core *self*, the person behind the actions—then stops right there, offering no avenues to change. You can tell it's negative and unskillful, by the way, because it usually contains some form of the verb "to be": *I* am *fat. I* am *bad at my job. I* am *a terrible daughter.* Such negative self-talk is paradoxically quite comforting sometimes. First of all, we've grown used to it. And secondly, it removes responsibility for changing behaviors. If you are, at the essence of your being, fat, then you might as well have another pile of deep-fried Kool-Aid, right? If you are, fundamentally, stupid, then why bother working on learning anything new?

Changing your inner script is not easy, and it will take constant vigilance. Please don't expect to be able to do it overnight, or even over the course of a year. The fact that it's a "script" means you're apt to stick to it. To go off script requires some uncomfortable improvising and ad-libbing. Here are four final pieces of advice about making those changes:

1. Resist feeling awkward about talking to yourself.

2. Whatever you do, don't criticize yourself if you find you have a negative script in your head. In other words, don't create a negative script about your negative script. If you do this, you miss the point entirely *and* compound the problem.

3. Whenever you talk to yourself, imagine you're talking to a person you love very much. To that person, you would always be supportive, nurturing, and gentle, even when you have to nudge in a new direction. Now, why shouldn't *you* be that person that you love? You might not think so right now, but I can promise you that you deserve it! It is of real, practical value to learn to like yourself, says the self-help guru Dr. Norman Vincent Peale: "Since you must spend so much time with yourself you might as well get some satisfaction out of the relationship."[10]

4. Use a loving friend or partner to help you determine
what to put in your new script. They love you for a reason:
Why? If you're uncomfortable receiving such compliments,
think about why that is and how that's serving you.

59. Do You Surround Yourself with Positive, Encouraging People?

PUSHING BUTTONS

To make this easier, let's spend some time talking about criticism,
and how the negative script gets into your head in the first place,
leading to the creation of all your "buttons." I have a patient, Lara,
who, while under my care, also received private counseling for issues
she had with her older sister, Judy. As an individual, Lara was very
well adjusted, showing maturity, composure, balance, and restraint in
nearly all areas of her life. But she really lost control around her sister,
who, not surprisingly, had an uncanny knack for pushing Lara's buttons. This scenario is not uncommon, especially among siblings. No
one knows our vulnerabilities and can get underneath our skin quite
as *skillfully* as our family members.

According to Lara, Judy's life was apparently littered with other
acrimonious relationships as well. Although I have never met her,
from what I could discern, Judy had many issues of her own to
resolve. However, by continually pointing out her sister's flaws, Lara
was diverting the attention she needed to examine her own role in
the relationship. Blaming other people, even if it is warranted, keeps
us from developing ourselves. Habitually, we protect our fragile egos
by pointing a finger at the other person, blaming them for the prob-

lems in the relationship, and this is not the way to skillfully manage a relationship.

Instead, when we're in a challenging relationship, we should also look at ourselves. If the goal is growth, maturation, and health, then it's worth asking: Why does it take so little for others to push our buttons?

While it's sometimes prudent to let go of a relationship, Lara didn't want to cut off her sister, nor was it realistic for me to expect her to do so. Lara loved her sister and wanted to improve their communication. But Lara's vulnerability to Judy's barbs pointed to a crack in her façade. Judy knew the location of this crack because she was there from the beginning, and might have even played a role in its formation. Rather than recommending she resist or deny the challenge posed by this relationship, I encouraged Lara to use it as a way to work on her own health, balance, and inner peace.

Together, we concluded that if Lara hit Judy back with barbs of her own, the divide between them would widen. Similarly, if she ignored the comments, that might paradoxically enrage Judy, who seemed always to be looking to get a rise out of her sister. Ultimately, all of Lara's pain in that relationship boiled down to her attachments and her ego. What was she willing to surrender? I reminded Lara that, at one time or another, we have all been hurt, abused, teased, and mistreated. From the earliest age, we're labeled: smart or dumb, energetic or lazy, popular or unpopular, exceptional or ordinary. Some of us are "odd" or "quirky," whereas others are simply "messed up" or "damaged." Often, these labels work in juxtaposition to our siblings (Annie is the "pretty" one and Nancy is the "smart" one). And frequently, these labels provide a mark or stigma that sets us apart from others, or connects us to undesirable or socially disagreeable characteristics. Every time Judy interacted with Lara, Lara had to face her labels in the mirror.

Lara's most sensitive label from Judy happened to be "bad hair." You can see how easily that label became a button for Lara. Judy frequently commented about Lara's hair, even though—or perhaps because—she knew that was her sorest point for whatever reason. But *why* did Lara have a button about her hair? It might sound overly simplistic, but once Lara let go of—or at least tempered—the issues surrounding her hair (her need to appear well put together and even glamorous), that button would disappear—and neither Judy nor anyone else would be able to push it any longer.

So I began by suggesting that Lara start the healing process by focusing on herself for a while and letting Judy off the hook for the time being. I wanted her to create some space, some time and distance away from the ongoing battle. This would be important before embarking on a new path that would require work of a highly personal nature. I reminded Lara about her ongoing work to build greater balance in her life and to reassess her attachments, loosening those that did not serve her. In this instance, she had to face that her vanity was one of her issues. It might have seemed cruel of Judy to always attack this one point of sensitivity, but it said as much about Lara: Judy was simply turning the mirror around.

I encouraged Lara to use Judy's provocations as motivation for her own personal growth. After ruminating about this topic over many sessions, Lara finally asked me, "How will I know when I'm ready to do this?" My answer to her was straightforward and simple: "When you no longer feel vulnerable to comments about your hair." That has so much more to do with Lara than with Judy. Ultimately, this is about self-esteem. And once we reclaim it, the negative script is erased.

EXTRAORDINARY HEALTH AND HAPPINESS

And so it goes. Until we address our buttons, the negative script will play on, and the button pushers will hold their magical spell over us. And when our buttons are pushed, our self-esteem will suffer. But, as we learn to live more skillfully, as conscious adults, we realize that it is we who are responsible for our own self-esteem and our feelings and reactions. Yes, it requires work, but so be it. It can't be achieved by swallowing more pills (even if they're prescribed), and it can't be bought.

Indeed, our health and happiness is not tied to how much we own and how much we control. In order to move toward the rewards of extraordinary health, you have to move away from the herd's suicidal drive off the cliff of material goods and false promises. Instead, you have to head in another direction altogether, facing yourself and actually committing to letting go of the negativity, ignoring the voices of the naysayers and those who would otherwise bring you down, serving their own self-interests.

What will really make you happy and healthy, if not a fancy car and a house on the beach in Saint-Tropez? You can start by cultivating a more positive mental state, which will have a positive effect on physical and mental health. In *Flourish: A Visionary New Understanding of Happiness and Well-Being,* "Positive Psychology" expert Martin E. P. Seligman collects some of the best data available on the positive influence on the health of things like solid relationships and a sense of life-purpose.[11] The best way to "build strength" against physical illness, according to the many studies Seligman performed or compiled, is—you guessed it!—to go well beyond the physical. In fact, after you correct for all the traditional risk factors for chronic diseases like cardiovascular disease (things like obesity, smoking, and high cholesterol), we find that positive psychological aspects, such as optimism, have positive effects on our specific disease states and our overall health outcomes—sometimes quite profound effects. These studies show that the right, positive mentality can help us with specific chronic conditions like obesity and diabetes, as well as with specific and integrated aspects of our lives, such as feeling useful and productive on the job or in the community.

OUR PARTNERS OF CHOICE

The fact is, there's plenty of science to support the notion that a truly integrated and holistic approach to health is the answer. However, the symptoms of poor health are most readily found by looking around at the faces that surround us at dinner. Our families and partners provide the best window into how we are doing. Thus, I'd like to take this discussion further to consider where we wind up once we leave our families of origin and how easily we can fall into the patterns of the past if we are not careful.

Think about it: we come out of our families of origin variously healthy or wounded, and then we find *families of choice*, the people with whom we surround ourselves—starting with our partners. Very often, as you've probably experienced in your own life or by studying those around you, we surround ourselves with those who fit the same patterns and fulfill the same roles as those from our youth—even when those roles are largely negative. Harville Hendrix, the psychologist who wrote the bestseller *Getting the Love You Want* and cofounded Imago Couples Therapy, sums up this phenomenon well: We sometimes seek in our partner the "imago" (Latin for "mirror image") of one or both of our parents, whom we perceive as having created a certain wound or series of pains in the way they loved us, or seemed to sometimes deny us or threaten to deny us love. The confusing and overwhelming experience of this all-powerful love of our parents— and the agony of feeling it slip away—creates an "emotional map" in us that we continue to follow into adulthood. We put ourselves back in the "same" relationship to try to heal those wounds. If we continue this way unskillfully, we simply relive, again and again, the pains of our childhood, and we never realize all the potential joys of our current relationships. Hendrix recommends a path toward bettering these relationships through what he calls "conscious partnership," in which we share with our partners those emotional maps, and help each other heal past wounds: "Happiness is *relational*."[12] It requires intimacy—opening up, even about your most "shadowy" past—with someone you trust enough to help you heal, without ever taking advantage.

So before I review the benefits of intimate relationships, it goes without saying that the most intimate relationship within your family of choice—the one with your spouse—can be either a source of terrible anxiety and pain, or tremendous support and joy. Take a good look at your present relationship, if you have one, and consider a simple question: Are you better off in this relationship or out of it? An unskillful relationship is a cancer that festers and swells, consuming your health and happiness, until the day it kills you. Like many, I know this from firsthand experience. Sometimes the most skillful decision is to recognize (preferably together) that you're no good for each other, and move on, letting each other go because you know it's the right thing. My former wife and I had some good years together and made three remarkable children. But it eventually became clear that we were not on the same page about how to work on ourselves and the marriage itself in order to maintain it. Our health on many levels was affected and hanging in the balance. Indeed, researchers have concluded that the emotional and physical stress of bad marriages can cause serious health problems. A good, stable marriage, on the other hand, promotes health and lowers disease incidence. One thing is for sure: hurting each other is not what skillful relationships are all about.

For a long time, common sense and anecdotal evidence led us to believe that people in love fared better in their health. Now research findings support a direct link between happy, stable relationships and better health. There are many examples,[13] and here's one that I think illustrates the point quite well: A long-term study of six thousand male and three thousand female British civil servants shows that healthy social relationships lead to better health, especially cardiovascular health, and unhealthy or negative relationships are often a key prognostic factor for myocardial infarction (heart attack) and congestive heart failure. The study showed that married women in unsatisfying relationships are *three times more likely* to have metabolic syndrome (a major risk factor for cardiovascular disease) than women in satisfying marriages. In men, marital distress is often associated with poor diet, lack of exercise, and substance abuse (alcohol chief among them), which might account for the higher instance of heart-related issues among unhappily married men. Both men and women in negative relationships are nearly *twice as likely* to experience a cardiovascular/heart disease event than those in positive, happy relationships. They are also more likely to develop depression, work stress, reduced self-esteem, anger, and a flat affect—which, in turn, are risk factors for any number of other major chronic health concerns. Yikes. Looks like you might want to put down this book and go say "I love you" to your neglected spouse. And for those of you without such a relationship, read on.

60. Do You Experience Intimate Nonsexual Relationships?

What exactly is intimacy? It's differentiated from other personal relationships by the presence of confiding interactions between partners. This is different from sexual intimacy, which is dependent on physical interaction. Either way, intimacy, at its core, is a social interaction. How does it work? Karen J. Prager, a family psychology expert from the University of Texas at Dallas, has studied the phenomenon: "Intimate relationships seem to buffer people from the pathogenic effects of stress,"[14] she writes, and "People who lack intimate relationships are at risk for a variety of ills."[15] Yes, love and friendship are good medicine.

Strong, intimate bonds between spouses have shown long-term benefits in helping cancer surgery patients recover psychologically and physically.[16] And research has also shown that intimacy improves the satisfaction of women during and after stressful events, such as pregnancy and giving birth.[17] Deep, personal relationships are indicators of well-being,[18] maturity,[19] and positive psychological growth.[20] Such intimacy should start early, with training from parents. Developing strong relationships during young adulthood leads not to dependency, as you might expect, but rather to a better sense of independence as we grow older.[21] High intimacy levels that start early also set us up for fewer psychological problems, such as alcohol and drug addictions, anxiety, and general mental and physical illnesses.[22]

Intimacy needn't take place only with spouses. Strong bonds between friends and family members can have the same positive physical and psychological benefits. One study shows that increased intimacy within a family, between parents and children, and between spouses, influences the mental and physical health of everyone in the group. The children in these families experience less mental and physical stress as they reach adulthood; they feel better, and they feel better about life.[23] This is important nowadays when most people in our culture don't get married until they're in their twenties, thirties, or older. That allows for nearly half a lifetime to practice developing "intimate" relationships of all kinds. It's difficult to start your experience of intimacy with your new spouse—you wouldn't know how.

Still, you needn't be connected at the hip to be intimate. Henri J.M. Nouwen, a Dutch-born Catholic priest, has written more than forty books about spirituality and relationships, often developing beautiful treatises on intimacy that I've shared with my patients and reflected on in my own life:

> *Intimacy between people requires closeness as well as distance. It is like dancing. Sometimes we are very close, touching each other or holding each other; sometimes we move away from each other and let*

the space between us become an area where we can freely move. To
keep the right balance between closeness and distance requires hard
work, especially since the needs of the partners may be quite different
at a given moment. One might desire closeness while the other
wants distance. One might want to be held while the other looks
for independence. A perfect balance seldom occurs, but the honest
and open search for that balance can give birth to a beautiful dance,
worthy to behold.[24]

The fact that the lovely metaphor above comes from a (presumably) celibate Catholic priest makes a valuable point for me: intimacy is not just about sex (a fact many men sometimes don't realize). If our intimacy is entirely sex-based, we'll find we have nothing left when we get older and our bodies stop working the way they once did. Even in the closest relationships, sex can be off limits because of age, health, or faith reasons, and intimacy can still flourish.

61. Is Your Sexual Relationship Gratifying?

Not to say that sex isn't important, if you want to have it! I've noticed in my practice that sexual challenges—clinical "dysfunctions" and general anxiety about sex—are a chief complaint and stressor among patients with chronic health problems. While I could engage in an intriguing chicken-or-egg debate about it, what's important here is to note that the free expression of sexuality is a sign of general health, well-being, and self-esteem.

I ask you if your sexual relationship feels gratifying because it's a good and simple measure of your ability to *open up*. As an apt generalization, health is determined in part by becoming "open" instead of remaining "closed."[25] The extent to which we're willing to be physically intimate and vulnerable is a reflection of the level of comfort and trust we have both with ourselves and with our partners, not to mention a good clue about our early lives (one of the places Sigmund Freud was prescient). If you have strong sexual inhibitions and aversions within your sex life with your partner; if you feel closed off, overprotective, or *too* vulnerable when you're naked or when your partner touches you, it's worth some reflection about where these feelings are coming from. People who've been wounded or violated—especially when the pain occurred early in life—tend to later protect their underbelly (both figuratively and literally), which often manifests itself in sexual hang-ups. Lack of comfort with sexual intimacy is a good mirror of our wounds in that general area. When we're wounded there—either by some past abuse, by something that happened that we consider shameful, or even by cultural mores and taboos—it's difficult to allow ourselves to feel sexually gratified, even if we want to. So we close ourselves off to these experiences, and this closure can block our connections to our partner and to others. Think about whether you're closed off in some way, sexually. Think about what you might do to safely, gradually, and appropriately open up, either on your own or with the right, trusted partner who can share that journey without ever pushing you too far, too fast.

SPACE IN YOUR TOGETHERNESS

I should mention again that although we are drawn together, intimacy does not require permanent merger. In fact, it's essential for partners, especially those who share a household, to give each other enough personal space, as this space helps each individual stay whole and fully available for their partner and the partnership itself. Relationships frequently fail because this principle is tacitly honored in theory, but seldom practiced. To paraphrase the brilliant Lebanese American poet Kahlil Gibran, the oak tree and the cypress do not grow in each other's shadow.[26] Instead, what we often see is partners subtly or not so subtly competing with each other: competing for attention, demanding that *their* problems be addressed first; suffocating their mate (and paradoxically, a vital source for their own nourishment). Those of you who garden have learned such lessons about how to sow seeds and tend to plants. We can apply the same lessons to our relationships. Says Proust: "Let us be grateful to people who make us happy, for they are the charming gardeners who make our souls blossom."[27]

Rabbi David Wolpe of the Sinai Temple in Los Angeles adds a spiritual component to this argument: "*Kadosh,* the Hebrew word for 'holy,' also means 'separate.' Yet *Kiddushin,* the word for the sanctification of marriage, also comes from the same root. How can togetherness come from separateness?"[28] The answer, to paraphrase the Hasidic theologian Martin Buber, is that love requires a certain amount of detachment.[29] This kind of holiness "is the dancing master of the heart: encouraging intimacy, insisting on distance, drawing close again."[30] Further, when we consider that the English words "holy" and "health" likewise derive from the same root, the circle is completed. Clearly the path to extraordinary health goes through our relationships.

So, why do we engage in such obviously unskillful interpretations of intimacy? Some people just seem incapable of leaving their partner alone. Their demand for attention is never sated, and they struggle when their significant other closes off in any way. Often, they react by drawing closer or becoming needier. Just as young children get attention from their parents by squabbling, acting out, or engaging in some manner of mischievous behavior, a needy partner gets attention and stays in focus by drawing negative attention. Many adults hold on to this behavior, particularly in their primary relationships, because it's how they learned to feed their ego or act in the presence of their imago. Yet even those who have insight into this aspect of their behavior appear to have little ability to do anything about it. Why?

Likely, the answer touches on their very primal fear of isolation or abandonment—part of that "emotional map" we form early on when we experience our parents' love, and fear that they will take it away. This fear overwhelms logical thought and supplants reason. In the context of a committed relationship, this behavior becomes pathological as one ego attempts to overshadow the other in a dysfunctional struggle for survival. Indeed, this competitive twist undermines the cooperative spirit of the relationship.

It's okay—it's even necessary—to let go a little. You must, or you will smother your partner. As Robert Brault writes, "There are days when you need someone who just wants to be your sunshine and not the air you breathe."[31]

It's also critical for you to have your own space, for both you and your partner (and the rest of your family) to help nurture your individualism and autonomy. This is one of the reasons that, no matter how much you love and adore someone, you ought not to make another person your purpose in life, your sole reason for living, your self. This is hard for a lot of people, especially women. It feels selfish or greedy or egotistic to think about and act on a personal sense of purpose that seems, ostensibly, to forgo the important people in your life. And, often, it seems impractical. You might wonder: Who's going to change the diapers? Who's going to worry about college tuition? Who's going to bring home the bacon and fry it up in a pan? I can assure you there's enormous room to accommodate the ones you love—but it's *your* soul and spirit, your life, your purpose, your health, your self, at stake. "Certainly your health and your body and *you* are more important than anything else in your life," say Rory Freedman and Kim Barnouin, the health divas who rocked the world with their straightforward *Skinny Bitch* series of books about women's health:

Yes, you have to put yourself before your friends, parents, boyfriend,
husband, and even your children. It won't make you a bad daughter
or wife or mother; it will make you a less resentful, more confident,
interesting, beautiful, patient, tolerant, and fun person to be around.[32]

62. Do You Feel a Sense of
Belonging to a Group or Community?

COMMUNITY CHEST

Now that we've explored our families of origin and our present, intimate relationships, it's crtitical that we take the next step and consider the larger context of our relationships, the groups and the larger community to which we belong—or ought to belong. We can't sustain extraordinary health in a state of isolation. There was a time not so long ago when it took a village to raise a child. At the least, many of us grew up in extended families, and many more in true neighborhoods, where people shared in the responsibility of child rearing and taking care of each other. But we've begun to look at the world through the unskillful lens of isolation that blinds us to the web of cause and effect. I propose that to be truly healthy, we must begin to take our collective interests into consideration when we make choices about our own health and well-being. We can call this "informed personal responsibility," a new kind of leadership that genuinely supports this notion of "universal health." Or we can just call it Skillful Living.

So, do you feel a sense of belonging to a group or community? This is especially important if your family of origin tended to hurt you rather than make you feel whole. We can go back to prehistoric times or simply look around at modern analogs to learn that we need each other to survive and thrive optimally. We need to feel that we *belong.* Do you feel part of your block, your neighborhood, your town, your country? In what ways do you express that sense of belonging, and how does it make you feel?

What happens in these groups is variously called intimacy, camaraderie, sharing, support, and so on. People stand by each other. People offer each other advice. People acculturate each other, accept each other. Paradoxically, we need others to make us feel whole as individuals.

In a formal way, we can join military or paramilitary organizations. We can join fraternities and sororities, political parties, or religious organizations. We can benefit from the strength of groups in less formal ways, too. We can belong to a poker game, a gardening club, a sewing circle, a choir, a cycling team—or even just a group of close friends who gather to travel or eat or shoot the breeze.

Lately, of course, many of us are joining social networks online. A recent study found that the average American user has 245 Facebook friends[33]—and some have many thousands. The total number of Facebook members—just shy of one billion—would make it the third most populous country in the world, after China and India. On Facebook and other social networks, we can reconnect with old friends, meet new people, share our latest triumphs and pains, and stay "connected" to others—or so goes the pitch. But there's a backlash against such virtual social networks. In a recent article, the *New York Times* highlighted the growing trend of smaller and smaller social networks. One social network, called Pair, limits each user to just *one* friend![34] Funny old world. Do you need a computer and an Internet connection to bond with one close friend? Is the next piece of advice from an ingenious computer company going to be "Turn off your computer and hug your spouse?" "We actually have to get together to make a relationship work," argues British evolutionary anthropologist Robin

Dunbar. Poignantly, he points out, "Words are slippery, a touch is worth 1,000 words any day."[35]

Yes, both literally and figuratively, the health benefits that arise out of group belonging are based on the fact that we can *touch* each other, hold each other and hold each other up, motivate each other, move each other.

Let me be clear about one caveat: yes, there are huge health benefits that involve our love of, and our cooperation with, others. I urge you to pursue those, but I warn you to be careful of the dangers of allowing others—either individuals or the masses—to overly influence your direction. This is a very personal matter. Remember, sometimes the herd is heading for a cliff. Where has simply following the crowd helped you so far in pursuit of either health or happiness?

63. Do You Go Out of Your Way to Help Others?

OUR BROTHERS' AND SISTERS' KEEPERS

Beyond merely belonging to a group, though, it's worth looking at what *you* can do *for* the group, for others, and the community at large. Do you currently serve others in some way? Do you volunteer? Do you go out of your way to give time or energy (not just money) to help others? Does the herd you belong to do any of these things? If you do, you're not alone. Every year, nearly 63 million Americans give of themselves through service.[36] Their dedication and compassion is a testament to the generosity of the American spirit. In difficult times, we come together to tackle our challenges instead of ignoring them. Lots of us face hardships today. But regardless of the severity of our present, personal problems, we can always find neighbors who are suffering more than we are—and whom we can help by donating our time, expertise, or goodwill. When we do something for others, we help heal them, and we help heal a hurting world.

Service opportunities "tap the energy and ingenuity of our greatest resource—the American people—to improve our neighborhoods and our world," according to President Barack Obama. Millions of citizens each year serve through Senior Corps, AmeriCorps, and Learn and Serve America. "We are building the capacity of organizations and communities to tackle their own problems by investing in social innovation and volunteer cultivation," says the president. And through United We Serve, a national call to service, the government is making it easier for women and men of all ages to find volunteer opportunities or create their own projects where they see a need.[37]

Look around—there's a heck of a need. Use your intuition and your senses to tell you where you can do the most good. Volunteering and altruism go hand in hand. According to C. Daniel Batson's book *The Altruism Question,* altruism is "a motivational state with the ultimate goal of increasing another's welfare."[38] It feels good, and you value it, but you do it for others, not your own gain. And no one forces you into it. The moment you engage in a behavior that promotes the welfare of others "without conscious regard for one's own self-interests,"[39] you're being altruistic. However, you don't necessarily have to think of it as self-sacrifice. You want to help others. But why? Why not just look out for number one?

Paradoxically, self-centeredness doesn't work for self-preservation. One study observed that the number of times a person used self-references in an interview (such as talking at length about themselves or using the first-person pronoun excessively) was an indicator of the extent of coronary heart disease.[40] We must think of—and help—*others* in our community to reap the beneficial health effects ourselves.

Research on the sociological and biological evolution of altruism suggests that our ancestors might have developed such altruism as a long-term survival instinct or strategy.[41] It makes sense that when you help the tribe, you help yourself. Further research proposes that the larger a society grows, the greater the inclination to share resources and labor within that group, especially when competing with another community.[42] This "pro-social" behavior eventually developed into the modern concept of altruism. One study observed that humans are unique in that "people in even very large societies also show strong tendencies toward altruism. Warfare, food sharing, and taxation are all examples of pro-social patterns of behavior that are common in human societies but nearly completely absent in other vertebrates."[43] Altruism and volunteerism are then beneficial to human society as a whole, but how does that affect smaller communities, and most important, individuals?

Well, researchers have found that "volunteers have higher levels of well-being and life-satisfaction than non-volunteers, suggesting that volunteering can play an important role in maintaining good health later in life."[44] This is true even when you're sick or suffering yourself. Another study found that patients actually experienced decreased pain and depression when they volunteered as counselors for other chronic pain patients. Somehow, dedicating themselves to others in their same predicament not only helped the others, but helped them, too. The study found that "making a connection" and "a sense of purpose"— two health factors we've already discussed—were major contributors to people feeling better.[45]

Psychologist Stephen G. Post, the author of *The Hidden Gifts of Helping* and *Why Good Things Happen to Good People,* writes that "positive emotions (kindness, other-regarding love, compassion, and so on) enhance health by virtue of pushing aside negative ones. . . . [They seem] to cast out the fear and anxiety that emerge from preoccupation with self."[46]

But it's important to note that this evidence is not just anecdotal. Altruism has physiologically measurable effects. One study describes something known as the "Mother Teresa effect." When a group of students watched a film about the altruistic acts of Mother Teresa, their salivary immunoglobulin A, a critical antibody, rose.[47] Immunoglobulin A literally provides a hedge against illness.

So take note—especially if you're a senior. Christine L. Carter, a sociologist at UC Berkeley's Greater Good Science Center and the author of *Raising Happiness,* writes, "People fifty-five and older who volunteer for two or more organizations have an impressive 44 percent lower likelihood of dying—and that's after sifting out every other contributing factor."[48] According to a study by the University of Michigan, volunteers with contributions of at least forty hours per year were likely to live a full seven and a half years longer than those who did not volunteer.[49]

We all need help and support sometimes for healing. But it's the act of *giving*—not receiving—social support that decreases the chances of disease and death in older adults, regardless of age, culture, social class, and gender.[50] The more you volunteer, and the more regularly you volunteer, the greater the chance that you will live longer. Just remember, though, that despite this knowledge, the healing effects of altruism don't work when you volunteer to help *yourself.* As one study reported, "Those who volunteered for self-oriented reasons had a mortality risk similar to non-volunteers. Those who volunteered for other-oriented reasons had a decreased mortality risk."[51]

It's never too late to get into the habit of doing for others. But, like financial investing, the earlier you start, the greater the rewards. People who were altruistic as adolescents grow up to have more successful lives—with better physical and mental health in late adulthood—than their peers who were not altruistic in adolescence."[52]

Keep in mind that your community includes more than just other people. Every day that you take care of a pet, you're volunteering and acting altruistically. You've heard this before, and it's true: blood pressure, heart rate, and mental stress all go down among people who own pets.[53, 54]

SERVICE STATIONS

In Rockland, the next county over from mine, there's a program called RSVP—Retired Senior Volunteer Program—based at SUNY Rockland Community College. It places hundreds of volunteers at more than 150 local agencies where they're best matched. RSVP's director, Gerri Zabusky (after whose name follows an alphabet soup of higher degrees), keeps it simple: "Volunteering is a noble gesture, and it has major benefits for the health of the volunteer."[55] I guarantee you there are programs like this one in your town or county—for youth, for seniors, for everyone.

So what can you do for others, and where can you start? Where can you feel a sense of belonging and/or contribute and serve others?

- **Your local volunteer fire department or ambulance squad**. You don't necessarily need massive training for this. They need drivers, "scene support" people, traffic officers, and folks to help with pancake breakfasts, fundraising, blood drives, and so on.
- **Your local library**. They need help getting donations and new members, stacking shelves, helping patrons, and reading to kids.
- **Your local community college.** They need volunteer tutors.
- **Your local pet shelter**. They need volunteers to feed, walk, and groom homeless animals, as well as raise funds.
- **Your local hospital**. They need candy stripers, clowns, and patient visitors.

- **Your local nursing home**. They need people to read to the residents, chauffeur them to appointments—and often just to sit and visit with them.
- **Your local kids' sports organizations**. They need coaches and assistant coaches, as well as team mothers and team fathers to bring snacks and equipment.
- **Your local veterans organization**. They need help writing to soldiers overseas, delivering aid to veterans, welcoming returning military personnel, and a host of other valuable services.
- **Your local literacy organization**. They need people to help kids and adults with reading challenges.
- **Your local Meals on Wheels or other meal-donation agency**. They need help preparing and delivering meals to the hungry in their homes and on the streets.
- **Your local church, synagogue, mosque, or other faith-based organization**. They need ushers, fund-raisers, cleaners, cooks, choir members, and day care and Sunday School helpers.
- **Your local Boys and Girls Clubs, 4-H, Scouts, Big Brothers/Big Sisters,** or similar organization.
- **My garden here at SunRaven,** or one closer to you.

All these places provide training. If you're willing to step up your volunteerism, as some of my patients have done, there are agencies like Teach for America, the Peace Corps, Habitat for Humanity, Doctors Without Borders, and others that provide high levels of training, a huge adventure for you, and an awesome opportunity to do massive good for others, assuming you can dedicate a large amount of time and energy.

But you needn't formalize your community service. Here are a few simple things you can do, starting today, that will take the focus off your problems as you begin to help others. This will help heal you both:

- Mow your neighbor's lawn
- Pick up the litter along your road (be safe!) or a local waterway
- Bring some food to an elderly resident of your town
- Clean up some graffiti
- Send a book or DVD to a soldier abroad
- If you see a soldier at an airport or restaurant, pay for his or her meal

64. Do You Confide In or Speak Openly with One or More Close Friends?

FELLOWSHIP

Beyond our original families, beyond our families of choice, and beyond the community lies another intimate connection: our true friends and fellows. Good health requires a level of intimacy with others that is similarly vital to our health and well-being. At its core, this type of intimacy is really about *trust*. Who would you call for a favor? With whom, besides your partner, would you share your most intimate thoughts? Indeed, since we often need someone to speak to about our partner, it is easy to see one example of how and why intimate friendship is so important. Therefore, it's essential to work up to trusting at least one other person in your life with confidences. This can be tough if your trust was broken in early life, but it's worth a try. You can start by always being trustworthy yourself. By listening attentively to friends. By supporting them. By never breaking their confidences. Be for them what you wish them to be for you, and they will be more likely to deliver. By the same token—especially if your trust and vulnerability have been violated—be careful whom you choose to take into your confidence. Make sure that person demonstrates the qualities of trustworthiness. Use your intuition.

You've heard the wise sayings: *Birds of a feather flock together. Tell me who your friends are, and I'll tell you who you are. He that walketh with wise men shall be wise: but a companion of fools shall be destroyed.* You know close friendships can influence you. But can they really benefit your health? Recent studies have shown that when it comes to physical and psychological health, close relationships with friends are as important as those with our families—and maybe even more important.[56]

One recent fifteen-year study found that Swedish men were more likely to contract heart disease if they lacked intimacy with close family and friends, and as well as if they lacked well-developed relationships within their community.[57] An earlier study conducted by the same researchers observed that lack of social support was one of two leading risk factors for heart disease in these middle-aged men.[58] Other research has observed that women diagnosed with breast cancer who did not have intimate relationships "had a subsequent 66 percent increased risk of all-cause mortality . . . and a two-fold increased risk of breast cancer mortality" compared to women who had close family and friends.[59]

Of course you know already that the effects of our social interactions can be either positive or negative. One thirty-two-year study found that "a person's chances of becoming obese increased by 57 percent . . . if he or she had a friend who became obese in a given interval," and that this influence extended to three degrees of separation.[60]

In the end, sound, healthy relationships are an indication that things are going well. On the other hand, unhealthy, dysfunctional relationships tell us that something is amiss. Simply stated, the quality of our relationships reflects how skillfully we are living. Good relationships require compassion, balance, flexibility, and equanimity. Our primary relationships—with others and ourselves—are a true reflection of our physical, emotional, and spiritual health.

PRACTICAL PRESCRIPTION 7: RECLAIMING TRUST

In order to foster intimacy and its associated health benefits, it helps greatly to be able to open up to other people and share your thoughts and feelings—in short, to be open to giving and receiving love from at least one other person. So I'd like you to identify a person in your life with whom you think you will feel the most comfortable opening up and sharing a little, or a little more than you have thus far. This could be your spouse, a trusted friend, or a family member. It could be a group in your community, such as a recovery group or a church group. Reach out to this person or organization, and tell them that you want to crack open the door of your relationship a little more. Here's the prescription: share your feelings about an important subject—one that you've never broached before. You needn't confess your most private and well-guarded secret (although you might find massive relief in that when you're ready); just share something that pushes your intimacy level a little further. This might be difficult. If you suffered horrendous abuse or for some other reason have a total lack of trust in others, you can write out these feelings in journal form, without ever having to show them to anyone. Use your intuition here. What would you like to share?

QUESTIONS FOR FURTHER REFLECTION

65. Have You Demonstrated the Willingness to Commit to Marriage or a Comparable Long-Term Relationship?

66. Have You Had Deep Tissue Bodywork or a Massage, and Are You Comfortable Being Touched?

67. Can You Let Go of Your Self-Interest in Deciding the Best Course of Action for a Given Situation?

68. Do You Have Regular, Effortless Bowel Movements?

At first glance, these questions might seem unrelated. But I assure you they're not. The issue here is how "open" you feel, how secure you are in your own space. Indeed, if you hold on too tightly, others, including the divine, cannot penetrate—and you'll be constipated to boot. Without getting too vulgar, our bodies are a clear reflection of our interior emotional and spiritual landscape. Extraordinary health is predicated on our ability to get so comfortable in our own skin that we feel safe being touched on the deepest level.

EMBRACING THE FUTURE: LIVING SKILLFULLY

I don't want to end up simply having visited this world.

—Mary Oliver[1]

69. Have You Conquered Your Fear of Getting Old and Dying?

WE'VE SPENT A LONG TIME TALKING about health, but we mustn't forget that integral to the process of life are sickness, pain, and death itself. It's not skillful in the least to pretend, as I've seen many of my patients do, that death doesn't exist, or that somehow you're exempt. Living with a *consciousness*—not to say an obsession or other form of neurosis—about death improves life and health. In fact, according to the eminent philosopher Jean-Paul Sartre, "It is only when we are aroused by our own deaths that the potential of our lives will become known to us."[2]

But it's important to note that you needn't—you shouldn't—wait until you're about to die to make your life worth living, to make it a "good day to die," as we've previously discussed. I'm afraid I learned this lesson the hard way, but I'm grateful now that I did. It's a painful story to recount, and a very personal one.

When I was twenty, a junior in college, I was spending the weekend away at my family's country home in upstate New York with one of my best friends, Brad, and his girlfriend, Suzy, as well as my first love, Mindy, the woman I believed would one day become my wife. While driving along a winding country road on a balmy summer day, our axle snapped, and the car flipped over numerous times. Mindy and Brad were killed instantly, and Suzy was horribly injured. Somehow, perhaps because I was the driver and had the steering wheel to hold on to, I walked away from the accident unscathed. However, the crash ripped my world apart. There I was one second with the windows down feeling the warm afternoon breeze beside the girl I loved, at the very height of my youth and hope—and one second later, it was all tumbling over the asphalt, landing in a heap of torn metal, glass, and the blood of the people I loved.

In an instant, I became profoundly conscious that I'd taken it all for granted. I realized I'd been living like one of those mythological princes I enjoyed reading about as a child—like Percival, maybe, from the King Arthur legends—a little prince forced out into the dark wood. And now, as I watched strangers cover Mindy with a sheet on the side of the road, I knew some cruel power beyond me had torn me from my fairy-tale childhood forever. It was already a mystery to me, seeming as dim and distant as that primordial forest. This—the hot pavement, the sirens, and the stench of gasoline—was the "real world" of which I'd heard my parents gently warn, a very mean place where love lies bleeding.

Chalk it up to youth or immaturity or the mind's inbuilt defense mechanism, but I was able somehow to shift my focus away from the awful loss, and on to more *practical* concerns. This is perhaps more common than you might think, I'd later learn. After the accident, I turned my attention to completing college and getting into medical school, which as you can imagine, takes particular discipline and hard work. Everyone said I was "well-adjusted, considering." I might have even believed it. After medical school, I started my residency at a prestigious medical center in New York City, and immediately following that became the training director of the program I had just completed. I was on the fast track. I was certainly a "survivor."

However, I found something amiss when I looked in the mirror: my heart was broken. I could picture it there, on the side of a Catskill highway still, where I left Mindy and Brad, who would never wear caps and gowns or get advanced degrees framed, who would never wear wedding rings or see their own children smile for the first time.

I was beginning to grasp in retrospect that I subconsciously chose medicine for a reason. And that medicine, too, was in a similar state, heartless and bereft. And as I began to inventory our parallel conditions, I realized with some horror that I'd *accepted* this state of darkness and incompleteness, both personally and professionally. Ostensibly, it was a successful career and life, but for me, it was a kind of self-imposed exile. I saw that I'd continued to pursue this, my childhood ambition, at least partially as a result of the guilt I experienced, feeling responsible for the lost lives of my friends. Perhaps on the plus side, the accident compelled me further into medicine, and a desire to save lives and heal hurts. But for more than twenty years, I lived in the shadow, not feeling worthy of coming into the light.

But, I did wake up with the recognition that my condition was compromising my new, even more important, role as a father. I worked especially hard to let go of all excess emotional baggage and transform any residual negative energy into something more positive, creative, and hopeful. I opened myself to the assistance of those who offered it—which wasn't easy. Doctors are notoriously bad at seeking help. And so are victims of survivor's guilt.

The gradual integration of my professional and personal life resulted in a more whole individual, and my path toward the light became clearer as I got a better glimpse of my life's purpose. I returned my focus to serving others, but knew I had to take care of myself to accomplish that. In order to truly take care of myself, I had to let go of much of my attachment to Mindy's and Brad's lives and the circumstances of their tragic deaths. I had to understand that people die, they move on, and as they do, they give us the gift not only of everything they taught us and shared with us, but something more profound, almost holy: they give us a renewed gratitude for our own breath, our senses, our time on earth. They remind us that our time is finite, but the resources we can draw on during that time are all but boundless. While my marriage didn't survive the fallout, my children are precious reminders of the potential for resurrection, and now I'm in love with the woman with whom once again I expect to spend the rest of my life. I'm no longer stunned and heartless at the side of that road, because I willed myself to turn and walk back into my life—because they loved me, and that's what they wanted me to do. And as I did, it felt as if they both climbed out of that wreck and brushed themselves off and, together, went the other way with equal hope.

I don't know exactly where they went, but I know it was a good place. And as I emerged from that darkness, and drew closer to my true calling, it was a good place for me, too. The universe conspired to bring information and people and resources my way. Indeed, as I began to write this book, the stories of the individuals I've included in the text came one by one, often in sequence, almost as if I was being channeled with the appropriate experiences to illustrate.

I don't want to dwell on the agony of that crash scene. But I want us to remember that such "accidents" leave an indelible impression:

they remind us of the certainty that *life can and often does change in an instant, a flash, the blink of an eye.* More than twenty years after the accident, I was introduced to the philosophy of Tibetan Buddhism, which stresses this same lesson. Buddhists maintain that while it might remain impossible to be *certain* about what happens after we die, there are only two realistic possibilities:

1. Either some part of us continues in some kind of afterlife; or

2. Nothing.

Therefore, Buddhists believe, quite pragmatically, that we should at least prepare for the *possibility* of Number 1. Something might happen in the afterlife. At worst, it's a 50/50 proposition. Sounds reasonable to me. Because if we assume there's nothing waiting for us, we might become more prone to lapse into a nihilistic existence, and give up caring about what we do and where we're going. We might wind up treating others and the place we all live like crap. This is not a "religious" chapter. But don't we have a shitload to lose if we choose wrongly, if we miss the point?

Indeed, I've seen this play out. As a practicing physician, I've been with people in those profound and meaningful moments right before death, hearing their last wishes and their final regrets. This experience, coupled with the accident that altered my life, compelled me to start living every day to its fullest and to teach others to do the same. So, in a way that might seem weird to you, but makes perfect sense to me, I've written this book with as much attention to your dying as your living—because they're one and the same if you consider them skillfully. Certainly, to deny the lessons in death by turning away is to give up the potential of life.

It hasn't always been easy for me to take this path, for me to help people understand the yin/yang nature of life and death. It required a lot of effort at first. Basically, I had to learn to express myself with even deeper compassion and empathy. I had to summon a great deal of tenderness and a delicate hand to connect to people when they were the most raw and anxious. I proudly confess I eschewed the advice I received in medical school to remain dispassionate and emotionally detached from sick and dying patients. I wept with my patients. I prayed with them. I laughed out loud. I still feel these patients' living presence and vital life force, which were so obvious to me when they were alive, lingering in my consciousness, having become, in some way, part of me, the same way I carry part of Mindy and Brad so many decades later. And some of them, like a patient named Steven, had such a momentous impact on my life that they fundamentally changed me as Mindy and Brad did.

As if on cue, Steven came into my life as I sat down to write this chapter, reaffirming how critical it is to live fully with every breath. More so, Steven proved to me that this process can work, that there is always hope, and until our last breath, joy can happen and healing can occur.

STEVEN'S FINAL CHAPTER

Steven's session began the way I start all my sessions, with the question, "What brings you here?"

And his answer was typical in many ways: "I have metastatic cancer, and I'm looking for something beyond conventional medicine to help me."

Steven was seventy-one, a domineering presence, a man who liked to maintain as much "control" over his life as possible. His considerable affluence allowed him to hire people to do his bidding. By his own admission, he was demanding, difficult to deal with, and nearly impossible to please. He often made the people around him feel they were never doing enough to meet his needs. I admit there were times I empathized with those people. Several of my fellow doctors had booted Steven from their care because of his demanding ways and unremitting self-destructive behavior. But I appreciated that there was more to him than what was on the surface, and I was willing to take him as he came.

Naturally, Steven tried to exercise the same dominion over his illness and impending death as he did over every other part of his life. While it was clear that he was not afraid to die in theory, he wasn't exactly keen on the gruesome particulars of the dying process itself, which, for him, represented the ultimate loss of his (illusory but all-important) control. So, he kept his focus on living, which was a good thing: he did everything possible to feel alive, every day he could. He could have hired a chauffeur but insisted on driving his own car. He got out of bed each morning and dressed himself, even when this and other mundane tasks that he used to take for granted became more and more difficult. He spoke of his desire to travel and shared his fantasies of making love to women again. It moved me that Steven never lost sight of living, though he was certainly coming closer and closer to death. Through it all it seemed that Steven wanted to *heal* his life—to become *whole*—before he died. I agreed to help him with this most noble and profound mission, even as I assisted with ways to ease his physical pain and stave off some of the ravages of his disease.

The details of Steven's illness revealed that his condition was rooted in his liver, the organ most associated with anger in many traditions, which was riddled with metastatic cancer (on top of his alcoholic cirrhosis). He had pages and pages of notes, in fact two giant loose-leaf binders filled with medical documentation, part of his efforts to control the illness. I mostly listened for the three hours it took him to review the history. But after all that time I responded with one simple question: "Steven," I said, "what are you so *pissed off* about?"

He was taken aback, I could tell, surprised by the "un-medical"-sounding question. But I could see he was holding back tears; my question had hit the mark. It seems that ten years earlier, Steven's ex-wife got a court order barring him from seeing his only child. The boy was now nineteen and had virtually no relationship with his father. Needless to say, Steven was extremely bitter, and very hurt. Yes, I needed to help Steven deal with the practical, "conventional" medical matters, and suggested some complementary treatments. But I also knew that in order to heal, he had to address his anger, which was literally killing him. He had no ambivalence about how essential that was, and I found him open to everything I offered.

I wound up seeing Steven every week for about a year. We went through the questions I outline in this book. We spoke of many profound things, the meaning of life and suffering chief among them. He began to resolve for himself one issue at a time. In an interesting way, Steven certainly embraced the idea that he was going to die. He planned his memorial service down to the finest detail, going so far as to compile a list of seven or eight people who would offer eulogies and writing explicit instructions for the orange ribbons he wanted distributed to the guests. He arranged the bagpipe processional, the music, the hymns he wished the mourners to sing. It was as though he wanted to really experience that service, and he got genuine joy, contentment, and peace from "playing it out" in his mind.

But he was still alive. And while he was alive, he vowed to tackle one challenged relationship at a time, calling on forgotten friends and even reaching out to some old nemeses for reconciliation. He really made a point of tying up loose ends. I admired him for that, and helped him whenever I could. Steven was a man on a mission, and was visibly excited as he completed each task. I was honored to be part of that process.

But throughout our time together, his relationship with his

estranged ex-wife and their son remained very much "unresolved," to put it clinically. Really, it was full of pain and regret. After we discussed this subject over a period of many months, Steven finally realized that the person with whom he was most angry was himself. Out of respect for his family's privacy, I won't tell you exactly why he was so angry at himself; it doesn't matter, really. All that matters is that as he came to this new level of awareness, he began to sense a deep course of healing unfolding in front of him. Though he had called both his ex-wife and son on many occasions, the conversations never went very far, typically ending in acrimony and hurt feelings. It was unclear whether they would ever forgive Steven for the slights they perceived, and he admitted it would be difficult for him to ever forgive his ex-wife for alienating his son from him. As he ruminated over the state of these relationships, his intense feelings and anger percolated, and, not surprisingly, his medical condition deteriorated. This is important: you often have to walk through the jungle to get to the waterfall. Steven was persistent and persevered.

Over the next several months, Steven reached out to his son more often, and with (what I believe was) greater and greater humility. There was a softening of their relationship and a developing rapport. Most interestingly, results from CT scans showed a coincident improvement and partial resolution of many of the tumors, even though he was no longer receiving any conventional medical therapy. Steven was noticeably stronger, getting out of bed more and dreaming once again of the ladies. He was more "present" in our sessions, and seemed more hopeful than at any time before.

Then, one day, his son called to say he was coming to visit! This was an incredible moment. I could sense the life returning to Steven. He immediately got on the phone and planned an excursion for the two of them to visit an old family friend in the Berkshires. He looked bright and animated. I was excited for both of them, and looked forward to hearing about their adventure when I returned from my own upcoming vacation. I had no reason to suspect that this would be the last time I would see Steven. He was as well as he had been for more than a year. Still, before I left that day, I was compelled to tell him how our professional relationship had become much more than a job for me, and he, much more than a mere patient. He had let me into his life in an intimate way, and this was an honor I didn't take lightly. Then, as I started to say that I was looking forward to seeing him when I returned, he interrupted with a foreboding tone to say he wouldn't be seeing me then. He was going to travel, he said, as he'd always wished. I had a peculiar premonition about that "travel."

And so it came to pass. His day with his formerly estranged son was indeed an adventure, and we never did see each other again. Steven collapsed while walking up the stairs to his bedroom just after he returned home from that healing trip with his son. He died minutes later. His final act, I'm told, was pulling out the endotracheal tube that the EMS team had inserted in an attempt to "save" him: Steven was ready to die, and did just that, with a smile on his face and his son in the room.

I don't tell this story to depress you—just the opposite! There are many uplifting and instructive lessons to be learned from Steven's story. First of all, both Steven and I were interested in the *sites* of his physical ailments. His condition started in his lungs, which are associated in many traditions with the complementary emotions of grief and courage—and the practices of letting go and moving forward, as we discussed in the last chapter. The liver, where his cancer took hold, is primarily associated with the energy of spring and new life and the emotion of anger. Indeed, the greatest challenge for Steven was to let go of this terrible anger and hurt, his compulsion to control, and to gather enough courage to confront his demons so he could effectively *transcend* his condition, even while it took an inevitable toll on his physical body.

The second interesting thing about Steven's story is how his body began healing as he started repairing his fractured relationships. So why did he die, and why wouldn't we consider his death a failure? And why did his death come just after the moment where he finally let go of the worst pain of his life? The fact is, I believe Steven was at a high point when he died, and this is a story of success. He'd suffered a long time, but in a way, he *chose* to die while he was still fully alive, when he had, like those medieval knights I worshipped when I was a child, fulfilled his quest. His quest was for forgiveness. His holy grail was his lost son. He rediscovered that lost boy after a very long journey. And he opened his heart and shared it with him, and vice versa. And with his heart open, he became more alive on that last day of his life than he had been for many preceding years. I'm certain he intended to leave his son with a positive image of his father, so the young man could move forward unambiguously with his own life, knowing he had been loved and missed by his father. And that he was a man who, despite deep human flaws, was worthy of love and forgiveness. I never expected to know what they said to each other—that was between them—but I was sure that in that one day, they went so far toward healing that Steven was whole (i.e., *healthy*) when he died.

But it turns out, I did find out! Steven's son gave the final eulogy for his father, which turned out to be a heartbreaking reminiscence of the day they spent together in the Berkshires. As I listened to Steven's son tenderly describe his father's delighted expression as they tried to evade security guards on the grounds of an old asylum onto which they had trespassed like boys, Steven came alive in my mind. I was struck with a profound sense that he was okay, that he had moved on now—in short, that he was in some kind of "heaven." His son went on to say that he was so grateful that in the last week of his life, his father was able to let go of all the things that had interfered so awfully with their relationship. They had come full circle, he said; what had felt like "work" for his whole life was complete now, and they were both free.

Plutarch writes, "The measure of a man is the way he bears up under misfortune." This to me is the most accurate way to measure the impact of Steven's life and all our lives. We're all going to have to deal with hardship and a measure of misery. Ultimately, we're all going to succumb. Who will we be when we do that? What legacy do we wish to leave? What impact will we exert on the ones we love? How will they remember us? I've been to scores of my patients' funerals and heard hundreds of eulogies. It's led me to the conviction that to live a life worth living, you should consider "beginning with the end in mind,"[3] as Stephen Covey proposes in *The 7 Habits of Highly Effective People* ("effective" and "skillful" are synonymous here): take a notebook and write out the eulogies you'd like to get from family, friends, and coworkers many years down the line when you die. Then go and live a life worthy of that high praise.

For me, I'd like people to say I was a skillful gardener. I sowed seeds in my personal and professional relationships that bore a lot of sweet and healthful fruit. I'm completely confident that what I offered Steven was life, and a connection to people, that extends today through his son. Steven made it through the jungle, transcended his past, and reached a new plateau, well beyond the limits of his physical condition. And, once again, his life touched mine and offered other lessons as well, concerning parents' relationships with their children and our culture's fear of aging. Let's discuss those.

70. Are You Willing to Learn from Children?

A few years ago, I was driving my then nine-year-old son Benjamin to the airport to go see his grandparents. Because he tended to get anxious about traveling at that time, we left several hours before his flight was scheduled for takeoff. Looking back, it was an unreasonable amount of time—four hours!—and it was a mistake, perhaps, for me to give in and enable his anxiety. What if he was bored or started to fidget? What if the amount of time we had to wait actually contributed to his anxiety rather than allaying it?

It turned out that because we arrived at the airport so early, he was a lot less anxious than usual, and that immediately put his daddy at ease. More important, we had the opportunity to talk, have lunch, and cuddle. It really didn't matter that we were at an airport or that we had to wait hours for his flight. At that moment, we were just present with each other and enjoyed ourselves by people watching, giggling at silly things, and marveling at the jets outside the giant panes. But the place and time were of no consequence, really. As he was boarding the plane, a thought crossed my mind. That was the best experience I had ever had at an airport. Although I quickly could have grown bored and restless, I was with someone I love, and the hours we spent waiting for his flight gave us an opportunity to spend time together. In retrospect, the "mistake" would have been to leave later.

I learned to simply be present in the moment, something most kids are better at than we adults. I got to see an airport, which I'd come to accept as a mundane and quotidian place, through the eyes of a child, for whom everything is still new and every day is an adventure. Recent studies show that infants' brains remain constantly lit up the way ours do only when we're experiencing those rare brand-new adventures. Of course! For a child, it's all new. I was reminded of this moment when Steven died. He got to spend his last day with his son—and that was a tremendous gift of renewal.

Could you find real fulfillment and joy by simply being in awe of a jumbo jet as a child can? How about by wondering at the cycles of plants and animals in response to seasonal and climatic changes to their environment the way kids do? My children and I used to spend countless hours sitting beside a small pond on our property, mesmerized by the iridescent quality of dragonfly wings. One early spring day, my daughter Caroline and I tried counting the many different shades of green we could see beside the pond (we lost count at twenty). These are the kinds of things that kids still notice—it's called visual acuity—but which we adults forget or ignore or deny, often because as we "mature," the ways we learn to communicate *limit* our understanding, rather than foster imagination and possibility. "Yes, *green*. I know what it is," we say. "The whole park is green." "Sure, spring. Buds and birds. Lovely." And then we go do our taxes.

Do you want to feel young and vigorous and excited again? Learn how to do that from the masters: your kids. Or somebody's kids. Offer to babysit. Help out with Sunday school. Volunteer for the Scouts or 4-H, or Big Brothers or Sisters. Do you remember that near-perfect moment in the 1972 film *The Godfather* when Vito Corleone, the murderous patriarch of the most dangerous family in America, spends his last moments with his little grandson, Anthony, in his tomato garden? Just before the Godfather dies, he's making the boy laugh by inserting an orange section in his mouth to form an exaggerated smile. The masterful scene (I don't know whether Mario Puzo, Francis Ford Coppola, Marlon Brando, or all three are responsible) is all about forgiveness, letting go, the cycles of life, reconnection to Eden, and making oneself ready for the transition to whatever comes next. After all the terrible things Don Corleone does in a lifetime of crime, he ends at peace, bringing joy to a child and feeling young again, in a place of growth and life. Often it is children, as was the case for Steven, as well, who bring us back to focus on what's really important.

LIVING WITH OUR EYES OPEN

The Godfather was ready to go, just as Steven was, in a way that's still difficult for me to grasp at times, especially when we're not talking about old men. Perhaps Mindy and Brad might have been ready on some level, too, but that remains a challenging thought. Still, we needn't understand this entirely. Indeed, it's easier to accept when our subjects are aged, having lived full lives. It seems fairer that way. But then others who have done just that remain unwilling, kicking and screaming along the way. Steven's story offers a strong message about placing the emphasis on living in the now, not on the imaginary monster up ahead, and goes on to show us that the concept of "anti-aging" is absurd on its face. Its foundation and justification is to protect us and save us . . . but from what? Death is completely natural. Avoiding it is therefore completely unnatural. Contrived and misdirected in this way, anti-aging efforts simply foster fear and create imbalance. And because the anti-aging mentality supports our desire to avoid confronting the very fact of our own mortality, the sine qua non of finding a meaningful life, in the end, it leaves us bereft and broken instead of whole and ready for the next plateau, as I believe Steven was.

In the end, we will reap the seeds we sow. Thus, if we cultivate a negative mind-set about death, which we do when we deny the significance of our impermanent state, then we will surely experience dread whenever we think about death. In turn, that will negatively affect our health. Alternatively, we can establish a brighter foundation on which to live and a more natural and healthful attitude toward the inevitable end of that life.

Unfortunately, too many people's lives end well before their physical body dies. And others wish to go on living forever, which is not the way it's meant to be. Instead, without becoming morbidly fixated on death, we need to look at it squarely and learn to accept it. With

clearer vision, we'll be able to embrace the journey and the transition. Only with our eyes open will we be able to see the challenges
as opportunities for continued growth. As long as we're growing and
learning and *doing*, we live. When we stop, we die. And that's okay, if
the time to stop is right and we've made that decision skillfully.

ACTION CURES FEARFUL AGING

This is not to say that we should ignore our physical health along the
way. Quite the contrary. But as I have been stating all along, taking
care of our physical health is dependent on our attentiveness to the
health of our mind and the attitude we maintain in living our life—
our relationship to all life and awareness of our greater purpose. But
it's also dependent on a healthy attitude and perspective with respect
to aging and death. Without that, we will suffer more.

Why wallow in fear of getting old and falling apart when we can
stack the deck in our favor by taking control of our physical health—
but also manage our state of mind, dealing with inevitable health
challenges along the way skillfully, meaning with foreknowledge and
the right attitude? The right attitude embraces the reality that we're
all human—and that state, by design, is ultimately fatal. There's a
cycle of life, and we'll move on our continuum until we cease to be,
to make room for new life, as Steven did, as happens in the garden
every autumn. As we mature and grow, we learn and expand; we
let go of unhealthy attachments, and we can experience more joy,
life satisfaction, and self-esteem than ever. Life should get better, not
worse—but it won't happen by accident.

This issue came into focus for me recently when a colleague introduced me to another physician, Paul, who knew a little about my
work and was eager to tell me about a three-year certified course
in anti-aging medicine he had just completed. Genial and eminently

likable, Paul seemed, at first glance, like the sort of person who could become a friend. He was convinced we would have a lot in common. I certainly respected Paul's knowledge, as well as his passion and genuine dedication to helping people live better. However, something about his approach put me off. So, in as tactful a manner as possible, I commented that it's interesting how much emphasis our society places on aging. It's even gotten to a point, I offered, where we no longer view aging as a normal part of life, but as a disease state. There is, in fact, now a specialty in medicine devoted to solving the problems associated with this "condition." While I didn't disagree with Paul's assertion that there's much to learn about healthy aging, I said the problem most of us have with growing old—isolation, fear, loneliness, lack of respect, and disenfranchisement from society—cannot be solved through a primarily technologically and physically oriented approach. He agreed but indicated that his training didn't cover that.

Indeed, unless we stop viewing aging as a problem that needs fixing, we might extend the life span itself, but this will have a mere marginal effect on the *quality* of our lives. If I could have prolonged Steven's life but had not helped him to heal his relationships, I would have only extended his suffering. Similarly, the billions we spend on vitamins and supplements, lotions and creams, plastic surgery and life-extension research will not ensure that we'll live well and die in peace, free of regret. Nor will the countless hours we spend building our physiques keep us from leaving a trail of broken relationships. From my experience, those who put so much emphasis on turning back the clock and prolonging their lives are going to wind up feeling terribly depressed and defeated when the realization hits that they have been fighting a losing battle. The intense focus, not to mention money, time, effort, energy, and thought, that we put into warding off aging offers us little insight into ourselves, or into how to develop anything other than our physical bodies.

We mustn't reject the wisdom that comes with growing old. The anti-aging quest robs old age of its inherent value and meaning. How have other cultures dealt with death? What does religion say? How does science deal with it well and poorly (i.e., what's the difference between helping your health so you can live better and trying to short-circuit nature by trying to live forever)? This question is likely on the minds of most of you. The "New Old," I've heard you called: the baby boomers. You're dealing with living longer, better, happier, healthier lives. But at the same time, as you get older, you inexorably will get sicker, eventually. The oldest of the nation's seventy-seven million baby boomers (those born from 1946 to 1964) are entering retirement—and more than ever are focused on proactive ways to improve their health.[4] Boomers are rightly worried. The years are catching up with you. In general, you're not taking it lying down. A recent Harris Interactive poll found that baby boomers are increasingly preoccupied with their health and wellness, with 73 percent of those surveyed concerned they won't be healthy during retirement.[5] The good news is, you're seeking out new and different ways to stay healthy and live skillfully. And your expectations are different from past generations. You *expect* to be healthy for as long as possible. In fact, your interest in staying healthy, coupled with your sheer numbers, is taxing the health care system more than any group in history. You represent the largest group of health care consumers in the country. It's clear that you and your compatriots are not ready to give up the fight.

Sure, you want to extend your life. I get it. As long as you're not simply interested in "life extension." Ideally, you're looking for "quality extension." What's the point of living to one hundred if your life is devoid of purpose, meaning, and emotional connections—not to mention if it's full of pain?

This is a fairly new concept in American culture. The Japanese celebrate a holiday called Keirō no Hi, or Respect for the Aged Day. The Japanese people take this holiday a lot more seriously than Americans take, for example, our Grandparents Day—just another Hallmark-enabled pseudoholiday. Did you even know we have a Grandparents Day? Know what day it is? Neither do I. But in Japan, neighborhood volunteers distribute free bento boxed lunches to elderly people. Smaller villages hold *keirokai* shows in which young people and schoolchildren perform dances and songs in a special ceremony for their older kin.[6]

In *The Gift of Generations: Japanese and American Perspectives on Aging and the Social Contract,* Akiko Hashimoto observes that an older Japanese woman's "adaptation to old age—and preparing for the likelihood of widowhood—has been deliberately planned," in contrast to an American woman's plans of "resorting to a nursing home as an eventuality that was wholly unanticipated and unplanned."[7] One way the Japanese do this is by building extended families, even sometimes informally "adopting" new surrogate children or grandchildren. Why are our cultures so divergent? Japanese culture has long revered the old, and it actively prepares people for old age. Only recently has America begun to plan skillfully for quality of life in old age. I want you in that camp. I want you to plan a little further than simply "I'll work until I'm seventy, then I'll retire, and then . . . well, who knows?"

71. Do You Actively Pursue Your Goals and Legacy, Even as You Age and Suffer Loss?

You probably all know people who worked actively their whole lives, then retired, and died very soon after. We must learn that a retirement spent in a rocking chair—with no goals and nothing to live for—will deliver death pretty quickly. Yes, you can relax a bit in your retirement, but I'd suggest some mission-based activities that fulfill and inspire you, some worthwhile challenges that take the long view instead of the short.

In short, we have to maintain desire, a *lust for life*—and we have to keep in the game, trying to better ourselves and our surroundings, rather than giving up or resting on our laurels, feeling that we've earned some rest. James J. Dowd, a sociologist at the University of Georgia, reminds us that we must continually and continuously work on bettering ourselves, fanning the flames of our passions, and continuing "to grow, develop, and learn about the world in which [we] live." Dowd argues, "It may be naive, idealistic, or quixotic, but behind many efforts of human beings to engage themselves in the world is the utopian wish to create, if not an ideal world, a world that is better than if we had not acted as we did."[8] It's *never* too late to think about this legacy. Never. It's just as important in maintaining a positive outlook as you grow older as it is when you're young and it seems your whole life is ahead of you, as surely Mindy and Brad thought up till the day they died.

To me, Mindy and Brad are immortal. Immortality comes not only from our own accomplishments and contributions, but also from our survivors and the following generations remembering and commemorating the things we did and the people we were, even long after we're gone. Your legacy and your life purpose can begin when you're young, as Brad's and Mindy's did. And it needn't be as universally profound as curing polio or walking on Mars. But, just as important, it should continue as you get older. Dowd recommends that you "undertake a challenge such as traveling to remote parts of the world, running a marathon, learning a new language, nurturing a new relation."[9] You can use retirement, the move to a new place, or even something as traumatic as the death of a spouse to spur positive change and a different outlook on life, writes Dowd.

Your legacy is your legacy, and while it might have been inti-mately tied to your spouse, one of you will likely die before the other, and the other will have to go on. I know it's tough when you're griev-ing, but studies show that if you can find your way to incorporate into the bereavement process *some* positive emotion—gratitude for the time you spent together, enduring love, hope, and so on—you're going to be more likely to survive intact, even more likely to develop long-term plans and goals. That means that a year later, you're more likely to come out of the process skillfully.[10] I've already mentioned that it took me much more than a year.

We're coming along to this kind of enlightened perspective on aging, but we're not there yet as a culture. According to a study origi-nally developed by Leo Srole and further developed by the renowned gerontology researcher Ethel Shanas, two-thirds of us still believe that "nowadays a person has to live pretty much for today and let tomor-row take care of itself."[11] I'm all for living in the present if it means letting go of past pain—but that doesn't mean we don't plan skillfully for a healthy future. So what can we do to prepare for it?

One key to quality of life in old age is taking care of your physi-cal body. You're going to die of something. Chances are it'll be heart disease[12] or one of the other Big 8. You *can* greatly stave off that inevitability by staying physically active—and you'll feel better for longer if you do. You don't have to run marathons: physical activ-ity will improve your mood and your vigor after just ten minutes, with progressive improvements over twenty minutes.[13] On a positive note, many boomers have already gotten this message. Did you know that boomers make up a majority of the membership of swimming, cycling, and running organizations?[14] If you're one of these active boomers, keep it up! But if you're on the couch right now, get up and read the rest of this chapter while on a treadmill or in a park you have to walk to.

Beyond physical activity, skillful eating also plays an important part in maintaining a healthy lifestyle long into old age. Here, we're not doing so well. Increased health and nutrition literacy is critical, especially for older men who are dependent on their spouses for knowledge of these two subjects. That means don't let your wife control your health—it should be in your hands. Researchers continually observe a phenomenon that we discussed earlier, that "many of the [older] men considered themselves to be healthy [even] if they took medications that alleviated symptoms or pain . . . a number of the men are taking a plethora of medications for illnesses and ailments" and "the cavalier manner in which these medications are taken is alarming."[15] To ensure not just longevity, but quality of life, we have to go beyond conventional medicine. It's not another pill that you need, regardless of what your doctor prescribes.

One recent study sums up everything I've been advocating: the key to skillful aging "can be defined as a balanced outlook toward old age—following the natural laws of one's body, maintaining tranquillity of mind, cultivating a sense of harmony with oneself and one's surroundings, and gaining the wisdom of handling challenges and thus making adaptations accordingly." The study, by sociologists from Western Washington University and Miami University, Ohio, calls this "harmonious aging," and it's very much in line with Eastern philosophy: growing old should be "regarded as a life stage that embraces both continuity and change . . . older people would define their meanings of life in terms of its own opportunities (such as spiritual growth) *and* challenges (such as physical change)"[16] (italics mine).

However, some of us need a reality check, which is part of the balance you need when considering aging and death. James J. Dowd points out that "desire needs to be regulated in the sense that it would be self-destructive to continue to desire to be able to do something that one is no longer capable of doing. Irreversible losses or impairments must be recognized and adjustments made." You must *reorganize* your goals and life plans following a life trauma or a medical impairment; by "resisting the expected tendency to withdraw from [your] usual levels of activity, those with desire will adjust, reformulate, and continue on with a new plan."[17] In short: Roll with the changes. Adapt. Move on.

And while you do that, feel good about yourself and your continued achievements. Research conducted in Hong Kong suggests that you should surround yourself with those who support you:

> *Older adults' self-affirmation of their strengths, aspirations, and more importantly their resiliency to isolation, rejection . . . and other adversities, such as not letting others look down on them, contribute a positive mentality that comes together, forming a "resiliency" to illness and other adversities.*

This study reiterates what we've already discovered: paradoxically, when things go wrong as we age—such as illness or the loss of a spouse—we should concentrate on the "possibility of converting negative experiences into impetus for generating resiliency."[18]

Study after study backs up this notion of resiliency in old age: "Sources of strength that turn out to influence positively one's sense of mastery include a positive perception of one's situation, openness about one's vulnerability and responsiveness to help." The key here is "openness about one's vulnerability."[19]

This reminds me of how my patient Steven handled the "death sentence" his doctors gave him. We'd probably agree that a metastatic cancer diagnosis is a real health crisis. In the Chinese language, the symbols for the word "crisis" translate literally as "opportunity riding on the dangerous wind." Therefore, every crisis is really an opportunity. They are synonymous. Learning to persist, evolve, and communicate effectively during a crisis is the essence of personal growth and Skillful Living. Steven was fortunate in a way. I'm certain that had he never developed cancer and faced imminent death, he never would have been motivated to heal his life and his relationship with his son. His physicians gave him no hope, which, paradoxically, turned out to be his greatest opportunity.

72. Do You Experience Feelings of Joy and Exhilaration?

Sometimes when I'm at risk of feeling discouraged, I think about Steven and his son running from the security guard that day at the abandoned mental institution in western Massachusetts, where for some reason those two chose to trespass. I think about the smile on their faces. The poet Rainer Maria Rilke writes, "All emotions are pure that gather you and lift you up; that emotion is impure that seizes only one side of your being and so distorts you."[20] People are moved and motivated by emotions. Just look at the common root of those words—*mot*, "to move." Life is a constant process of moving in the direction of satisfying emotional needs and wants. Why are our emotions, or feelings, so important to our health? Positive psychology researcher Barbara L. Fredrickson argues, "The capacity to experience positive emotions remains a largely untapped human strength. The possible benefits of positive emotions seem particularly undervalued in cultures like ours that endorse the Protestant ethic, which casts hard work and self-discipline as virtues and leisure and pleasures as sinful."[21] Get over that! Positive emotions are the health gifts that keep on giving. Positive emotions, if you know how to tap them skillfully, can and will lead you toward extraordinary health: they will make you feel better, and they will make you more psychologically and physically resilient in the face of life's challenges.

There's an evolutionary basis for the benefits of positive emotions: Fredrickson notes that our ancestors used them to build "their personal resources, including physical resources (e.g., the ability to outmaneuver a predator), intellectual resources (e.g., a detailed cognitive map for wayfinding), and social resources (e.g., someone to turn to for help)."[22] We build these resources when we're safe and secure, and we can turn to them when things are bad, as they surely will be, occasionally. It's only when we are feeling *excessively* or *inappropriately* bad—stressed, angry, frustrated, hateful, and so on—that we see short- and long-term individual and societal ills resulting. These problems range from anxiety disorders and depression to heart disease and cancer. Norman B. Anderson, author of *Emotional Longevity,* enumerates what he calls "the big three" of negative emotions: "sadness/depression, fear/anxiety, and anger/hostility." It's not that these emotions, although negative, are "useless or should be avoided." They have their place. It's only when we experience these negative emotions all the time and whole hog, unskillfully, that they can have "profound consequences."[23] We've seen a lot of evidence already that, as author Stephen G. Post puts it, "the consequences of these negative emotional responses are increased susceptibility to disease and worse health outcomes"[24]—not to mention their negative effects on the quality of our life today.

But it works the other way around as well: you can channel positive emotions into an effective prevention, coping, and treatment plan for counteracting depression and other negative feeling states. Simple, regular happiness might not cure disease, but it looks like it can protect us against illness and disease in the first place,[25] even in old age.

So get happy about something. Get genuinely interested in something. Better yet, get genuinely excited. What do you have to be happy about? How about your job? Your hobby? Your kids and grandkids? Your health? Your pets? Art? Nature? Music? Friends? Politics? Okay—maybe not politics! But there's a world of possibilities out there if you open yourself up. Whenever I see my chickens and their new babies running around the yard, I feel joy. Whenever I see my patients smiling. Whenever I taste great homemade cheese. I could write a whole book about the stuff that makes me happy. You could, too.

Sustained excitement and joy will entice you to continue to explore, grow, and learn. These are all fun things, but they're also necessary for survival—the longer you maintain them, the longer you're likely to live, and the happier and healthier you'll be as you live. And the better you'll be able to cope during the inescapable bad times: *resiliency*. The resources you'll develop, Fredrickson points out, become "durable resources that can be accessed in later moments, and in other emotional states."[26]

You don't have to jump off waterfalls or go skydiving to experience exhilaration and joy. Simple physical activity can do it, because it allows us to experience catharsis for our anger and hostility—emotions that might otherwise be directed toward the self in the form of depression,[27] while at the same time releasing endorphins and other feel-good hormones. And here's something interesting: a recent study observed the benefits of simply *writing* about positive and exciting experiences, which "enhanced . . . positive mood" and correlated to generally better health than those in a control group.[28] No wonder I've felt so good while writing this book for you! Why don't you start a journal today, and write about what makes you happy.

The resiliency-causing emotions, joy and exhilaration chief among them, as well as the fear-slaying positive outlook required for skillful aging, all come down to one factor: your willingness to see life, even the end of life, as a great adventure worth undertaking with vigor and enthusiasm, as Steven did deliberately, and as

Mindy and Brad did serendipitously, just because they were young. Participating in and having a sense of adventure (such as kayaking or hiking) benefits "character development such as self-esteem, determination, dependability, ambition, and independence,"[29] according to researchers in the field of "adventure education." An adventurous life helps with overcoming fears, enhancing the ability to cope, the opportunity to experience new activities, increased compassion and respect for others, and better self-expression and communication skills.

But adventure's not just about kayaking and skydiving or even physical challenges at all. People experience individual adventure in multiple ways.[30] It's about challenging *yourself,* whatever that means. Maybe it means joining a choir, building a birdhouse, or trying an online dating service. I've been thinking about planting some new crops in my garden this year: that'll be an adventure. Adventure is about doing new things regularly. It's about your spirit, which we've learned is inextricable from your well-being.

At its heart, embracing the adventure of the life you've been given is tantamount to finding the elusive "meaning of life." In *Emmanuel's Book: A Guide for Living Comfortably in the Cosmos,* authors Pat Rodegast and Judith Stanton share wisdom from Emmanuel, a symbolic name for a powerful spirit they "conversed" with: "The purpose of life is exploration. Adventure. Learning. Pleasure. And another step towards home."[31] I believe these wise words could provide the basis for our common understanding of the meaning of life and extraordinary health. I have seen in my patients and in those to whom I regularly speak a hunger to explore this and other critical questions posed in the quest for Skillful Living.

73. Is Your Outlook Basically Optimistic, or Can You Envision Yourself as More Optimistic?

74. Are Playfulness and Humor Important to You and Do You Have a Sense of Humor?

In the 1997 Italian film *Life Is Beautiful*—based on a true story—a Jewish waiter played by Roberto Benigni literally laughs and jokes his way through the nightmare of the Holocaust. He's not crazy. He does this for the sake of his loved ones, especially his young son. He convinces his son that the concentration camp is just an elaborate game in which the quietest, least-complaining boy will win a new tank. How could anyone maintain humor and tenderness in the face of such unspeakable horror? Simply, he chooses to create for his son an alternate, more optimistic reality, one that is necessary for the boy to endure in order to survive the hellish conditions. If he cannot overcome his situation, he has to create a new one altogether.

History is full of such hopefulness in the face of horror. A group of Tibetan lamas (Buddhist monks) who were imprisoned for years in a Chinese gulag realized through meditation that their confinement was an opportunity for personal and spiritual growth. The lamas were so appreciative of this "opportunity" that they sent a thank-you letter to the Chinese government. They literally found, as a friend of mine observed, "freedom in confinement." Now *that's* optimism!

Every day we see examples of people who are impoverished in some manner but whose lives are nonetheless filled with beauty, contentment, and peace. On the other hand, how many of us are relatively well off in the world, but wallowing in misery? To see which side of this equation you fall on, look in the mirror. Listen to the script in your head. Listen to yourself as you speak to your friends or think on your drive home. Reread your Facebook posts for the past year. Who is that person that is you? Is she grateful—or resentful? Joyous—or bitter? Hopeful—or hopeless? Thankful—or ignorant of the bounty around her? Free—or "imprisoned" by circumstances?

If you don't consider yourself an optimistic person, can you at least find a part of you that might still have the *capacity* for optimism? A hint, at least, of the desire to rise above your condition? If you have any doubt, I suggest that you don't give up. Yes, you will likely discover that you cannot change certain things in your life, such as your job or difficult family member. But, as James Baldwin writes, "Not everything that is faced can be changed; but nothing can be changed until it is faced."[32] So really look in the mirror and focus on what you *can* change. That can start with your attitude. Your beliefs. Your perspective on yourself and the world around you.

It won't happen instantly. Optimism is a muscle. You have to flex it if you expect it to get stronger. So start off small. You can certainly resolve to eat more skillfully, to get more in touch with nature, to drink more water, or to reconnect with a long-lost friend or relative. You can resolve to be kind, empathetic, and compassionate in your dealings with others, perhaps especially that recalcitrant relative. You can pay attention to your senses. You can cultivate a purpose for your life, and act on it. You can let go and forgive. You can be for someone else in your life a model for this kind of extraordinary health.

At the least, learn to laugh at yourself and at life. There's no need to be so serious.

PRACTICAL PRESCRIPTION 8: FOLLOWING YOUR OWN ADVICE

Each of us has wisdom and experience worth sharing. How many times have you provided good counsel to your friends, relatives, children, clients, coworkers, or employees? Now it's time to do this for yourself—to follow the advice you so eagerly give to others. You've gotten to this point in the book, so I'm certain you're more in touch with who and where you are in your life than you were when we began this journey. Remember, I might be the doctor, but you're the greatest expert about your health.

After reading this book, you might feel especially prepared to offer others advice. As important, I hope you will find that you are in a better position to take care of yourself first. Now is the moment of truth. Now is the time to break through and release the habitual patterns of thinking and behaving that no longer serve you.

Try the following exercise, which I developed along with my sister, Deborah, after some trying times. Starting today, then every few months or so, write yourself a letter full of wise, personalized advice, just the way you might write to a beloved friend. Don't preach, though. This letter should be loving and conversational, gentle and compassionate. It's important to avoid the overbearing, moralizing tone that usually provokes denial, ambivalence, and rebellion. This letter should be conversational. Here's a brief example one of my patients shared with me:

Dear Darren,

I hope you're well. I'm just writing to give you some advice, which I hope you'll take in the spirit in which I intend it: love and respect. I've noticed lately that you're getting down in the dumps about the twins moving out. I've noticed you haven't done much more than watch TV for a few weeks when you get home from work. I know you're not happy about this. I have some ideas. Sure, you're sad about the empty nest, but what about concentrating on those eighteen amazing years you all got to spend under one roof? What about remembering that time the girls tried to build that tree house and found the cardinal's nest? Or the trip out West when everyone got carsick together after all those doughnuts? And how about this: How about letting that pride swell inside you that both girls got into great colleges, and even got scholarship money? You know how much a part of their development you played. How about focusing on the joy you feel that they're starting their exciting lives now, full of possibilities? Before you know it you'll be shaking hands with promising young men in tuxes, and then, the babies will come! But, meantime, I've got some more advice, too: How about now that you're alone with Diane, you work on some of that stuff that's been bugging you all these years? How about being more attentive? How about getting more involved in her volunteer work, as she's been hinting at? How about getting intimate more often, and more spontaneously? How about you finally let yourself spend some time and energy on you—your health and future? How about it, Darren? I think you're totally worth it.

Love, Darren
P.S. You could stand to put down the Twizzlers, man!

QUESTION FOR FURTHER REFLECTION

75. Do You Feel a Strong Need to Be Right or in Control?

Well, what if you're wrong? What if the paradigm you have subscribed to is off base, and all your "rules" are misguided? Not possible? Are you *that* sure? This is a question that asks you to consider a more humble approach to living, and the possibility that there's something more you can learn that will ultimately prove beneficial. I'm not suggesting that you toss out all that you believe in. I just want you to consider how things might be different if you let go of your attachment to other people's points of view, in particular. In the end, the test is, are you thinking for yourself?

9

TAKING THE LEAP TOWARD EXTRAORDINARY
HEALTH: MOVING FORWARD

*Creating a new theory is not like destroying an old barn and
erecting a skyscraper in its place. It is rather like climbing a
mountain, gaining new and wider views, discovering unexpected
connections between our starting point and its rich environment.
But the point from which we started out still exists and can
be seen, although it appears smaller and forms a tiny part of
our broad view gained by the mastery of the obstacles on our
adventurous way up.*

—Albert Einstein[1]

76. Why Do You Have the Symptoms You Have Now, and Why These Specific Symptoms?

THROUGHOUT THIS BOOK, I'VE SHARED WITH YOU some of
the fundamental questions that underlie the slow medicine path to
extraordinary health: Skillful Living. And, rather than answer the
questions for you, I've attempted to walk you through the process of

asking yourself these questions and helped you to think about—then
gradually act on—the answers you come up with:

- We've learned that when we live skillfully, we're not
  always trying to *control* things.
- We've learned that it's best to act in *alignment* with natural
  rhythms and cycles.
- We've learned to view the body not as a series of
  autonomous parts, but as a *whole* entity, inextricably linked
  to the elements of our mind and purpose that embody us
  as whole people.
- We've learned that *no man is an island.*
- We've also learned that past hurts can continue to
  adversely affect our health if we don't *let go and rebuild.*
- Ideally, we've learned to be more *present* for the things in
  the present that really matter—like our relationships.

I trust that you've come to understand by now that these factors—
and not the "absence of disease"—constitute the fundamental nature
of extraordinary health.

Now, at this point I'd like you to begin thinking about two last
important questions: Why these symptoms? And why now?

As I do with the patients who visit me at SunRaven, this is when I
ask you to restate and reframe your health challenges and your health
objectives. Often they're quite different from when our consultation
began. I find that a good place to begin this final chapter of our consultation is to make sure you have a better understanding about why
you have the symptoms you have *now*—and why you have these *specific*
symptoms to begin with? After reading through the previous chapters
and considering all of the yes/no questions that preceded this one, it's
now a good time to consider the *context* of your quest for health. The

questions here are, Why do we get sick? Why do we find ourselves with certain ailments and challenges in the first place?

I'm hoping this question might appear less esoteric—you know, "out there"—now that you've gotten this far in the process of Skillful Living. There's nothing more concrete than understanding the relationship between our life and the circumstances we find ourselves in, health-wise. Viewing life and health holistically, as we've come to learn, requires that we look for unifying themes that connect all the dots, across all the aspects of our lives. Essentially, this question might provide the most significant clue yet, indeed the key that breaks the code and solves your most challenging health riddle. But to get at it, we have to leave the Western medical paradigm once again, and consider the knowledge and wisdom that's accumulated through thousands of years of humanity, before the microscope was even imagined. We've got to look in that mirror again, and once again tap our intuition.

There are two parts required for this decoding process. The first is to understand the *timeline* for the development of your most important and pressing symptoms: When did your symptoms first appear, and in what form? What was going on in your life during that time, or immediately preceding it? Just think about how helpful this was for Steven. Indeed, it opened the door to his eventual recovery.

Here are some examples from other patients I have seen recently. Note how the associated issues didn't always appear obvious at first, but in each case there was definitely something going on:

- I got an annoying rash behind my knee. It started in 2004. This was right after I got laid off. It spread around my left leg within a few months. It was ultimately diagnosed as psoriatic arthritis.

• Once we moved to the city, I started to get tired all the time. Within a year, I was missing a lot of work, and even family events. They gave me antidepressants and did all kinds of tests but never really diagnosed the problem. Now I'm barely keeping it together. When I go back home to the farm, though, I definitely feel a little better. I wish I could stay there longer.

• I don't know whether it's migraines "officially," but I get really bad headaches at least once a week. I can't even *think* when they're happening—they knock me on my butt. I guess they started a few years ago. Everything was going fine then—and still is: I'm a very successful lawyer, always busy, always traveling, and often in the limelight. I love what I do—especially being able to help desperate people. One thing I'm not crazy about is that I'm not able to be around my family enough. But then other times, it aggravates me that they're too demanding. What do they think pays for our house and summer camp and great vacations?

• My doctor tells me it's a typical pattern: First I gained weight in my thirties. I got high cholesterol and went on a drug. My blood pressure wasn't so hot, so she put me on another drug. Then my blood sugar went up, and I started to take a third pill. That didn't work, and eventually, I started a few shots of insulin. Still getting fatter for sure, and not exactly feeling great about my health. What was going on when all this started? Nothing, really. When I was twenty-eight, I lost my job, and that was awful, but I'm not going to say that *caused* any of my symptoms. In fact, to be honest, it was a bit of a relief: I hated that job. I think it might have been the stress of looking for a new job—which lasted two years—that did me in.

• I know what's going on. It's the whole priest sex scandal thing. When all that hit the news back in the eighties, it freaked me out. I wished no one would talk about it. I felt like every time it came up—whether someone was talking seriously or making a joke—they could see right through me to my secret. I thought about it *all the time*. I was literally losing sleep. I was clenching my jaw. And then I could tell that I was getting physical symptoms: terrible diarrhea, and my stomach was always cramping up. For a while there, I was actually bleeding in my stomach. I think it was all that stuff that happened when I was six, trying to get out.

The idea here is to look into what was going on in your life when your symptoms began, to recognize the initial trigger of the "imbalance" that caused your health problem. What did those triggers represent? Was it loss? Trauma? Overthinking? It's basically self-therapy (though if you prefer, you can do it with a trusted professional). Finding your triggers can help you avoid them; you can begin to regain the original state of balance that kept the symptoms at bay. For example, if some great instability occurred around the same time your back began hurting, reestablishing stability now can shut down any recurrence of the trigger and go a long way to lessening or preventing symptoms. It might take some time—and cause some unpleasantness—to go back and figure out what was going on in your life that might have triggered the onset of your symptoms, but it's a worthwhile endeavor if you want to achieve extraordinary health.

Look at it this way: You wouldn't treat the pain and inflammation of a splinter without first removing the trigger—the splinter itself—

and ever expect to get better, would you? You could keep applying Band-Aids and ointments, and taking lots of pain pills, but until you deal with the trigger, the pain will persist (and, eventually, infection will set in). I realize as I use that example that it's not entirely accurate: the truth is, the body itself understands this dilemma, and it will work hard to eject the splinter on its own. But if you keep jamming it in, you'll defeat that self-defense mechanism.

THE MIND-BODY CONNECTION

The second part in this process is to delve more deeply into the association between the physical *site* of the first symptom and the mental/emotional *state* that's related to it. For example, I've seen in hundreds of my patients that the lung and colon are likely associated with the emotion of unremitting grief—the prolonged attachment and subconscious desire to *hold on,* which we discussed in chapter 7. Similarly, we know intuitively and from personal experience that the head, neck, back, and shoulders are associated with mental and emotional stresses, and so on. While there are a few physiological causes of pain and inflammation in those areas, it's much, much more likely that the trigger, as we're defining it here, is emotional. This is especially true when the condition is a chronic one. In fact, I've seen countless times that when my patients get at the root of underlying *emotion,* their chances for physical relief become far greater. And this is well documented in the recent literature. Moreover, there are dozens of traditions dating back thousands of years—from traditional Chinese to Native American medicine—all of which focus on these associations between parts of our bodies and the emotional state to which they are linked. In each of these divergent cultures, the map of connections is quite similar, giving it a fair amount of credence in my mind. Find a healing tradition that suits you and explore the connections.

The goal for you is to understand the particular ways your body and emotional states are connected, and to work toward ways to reduce your physical susceptibility to the imbalance that results from those states. Sometimes, just learning to recognize the triggers will stop the emotional states. But often, you will have to learn creative ways to avoid them. You can employ techniques such as simple forgiveness, to "let go" of the trigger. To borrow a metaphor from the genetics versus lifestyle debate about health, a gun might pose a *potentially* deadly threat, but it can't fire on its own. *You* have to pull that trigger—or holster the gun.

So my suggestion here is to stop putting patches on those recurring splinters and work on ways to prevent them from getting under your skin in the first place. Get a journal or a notebook and write down your main symptoms. Maybe you can do this as a timeline. Then write the major life events that correspond to the periods when the symptoms began, and when they flare up. You can think of those circumstances as the initial triggers. Are symptoms still associated with the vestiges of those triggers? Do symptoms flare up when those subjects come up? Surprisingly, it's often that simple. Next, see if you can identify the *emotional states* associated with both the life events and the health symptoms on your health timeline. Remember the equation:

> **TRIGGER** (life circumstance) ⟶ **EMOTIONAL STATE** (the feelings it brings up) ⟶ **CHRONIC SYMPTOM** (in the body site where the emotional state manifests) ⟶ **ILLNESS** (the systemic problem associated with the symptom and site over time)

I have seen people who've suffered their whole lives from debilitating symptoms like headaches—who have taken dozens of drugs and tried scores of treatments unsuccessfully—virtually cure themselves of their ailments by going through the process of mapping their own equations. Here's how two patients, Connor and Dawn, summarized their efforts:

> • I was always looking for food triggers like MSG and sulfites (or lack of sleep or exposure to light or whatever) for the cause of my migraines. But when I did the timeline and kept a log, I figured out that they seemed to first come on when I was still living with my parents and times were tough at home. I spent a few months continuing with the journal and realized that I often got migraines soon after I talked to one of them on the phone, or even when I was just *thinking* about them and all our "issues." (I also learned from a food diary that I get migraines a day after I eat chocolate.) Don't get me wrong; I love my parents. But as I kept going with the log, I figured out that even when something was going on with them that was just *on my mind,* a migraine would follow, within a day or two. That was freaky. But why was it happening? It took a year, but I got to the bottom of it, a pretty deep well of anger and resentment. The short of it is this: My brothers got a free ride, but I caught hell from them, always. I couldn't do anything right. Once I started to talk about this—with my brothers and friends, and eventually with my parents—the headaches started to get much less frequent. Like you said, I was able to "let go" of the emotion, so my body let go of the illness. And I got better able to sense my trigger emotions, so I could work on keeping them in check. My headaches are 90 percent gone now, and that's dramatically improved the quality of my life. Not to mention my relationship with my parents is much better—more honest and more forgiving. Man, I miss chocolate, though.

• I don't perfectly understand why my knees and my other joints are associated with fear, but I had two problems for a very long time. All my joints ached like hell, especially my knees—and I was constantly afraid they would give way when I did any kind of physical activity. That wasn't the only thing I was afraid of. My friends always said I didn't try new things, and they were right. This all started in childhood, which is a long story—a pretty crazy-looking page on my timeline—but suffice to say I learned pretty early and pretty painfully not to take any risks at all. To summarize, when I was eight, we were at the beach, and I swam too far out, and got caught in a rip current. I was swept miles down the shore before I was rescued, exhausted and nearly drowned. I had to spend the night in the hospital. But my mother was nearly committed herself, she was so crazy over it. My parents became overprotective, and I suppose I followed suit. Total paradox, but following your suggestion, I tried treating the *fear* first, instead of the physical symptoms of joint pain. I read somewhere that "action cures fear"[2] so I tried to take some action. It didn't make any sense to me at first, but when I pushed myself, like when I decided to go hiking with friends, my knees felt better than they do when I'm just walking around a grocery store. After a while, when I stepped it up—I did a ten-mile hike, eventually, *alone*—each mile marker I passed gave me more self-confidence, and less pain. Hiking on my own, especially in new places, gave me all kinds of self-assurance. I applied for a promotion and got it. I asked my boyfriend to marry me, and he said yes. I was finding that taking chances was making me a lot less afraid, and—very weirdly at first—the pain in my joints *almost* disappeared. What's interesting now is that I don't consider it weird anymore. Whenever I feel pain in my knees the first thing I do is look at the stuff going on in my life and my emotions about it. I always assume that's the cause.

This "context" equation of triggers, emotional states, symptoms, and illness isn't weird at all, as Dawn discovered by mapping her time-line. It's the essence of integration, the basis for genuinely *integrative* medicine.

PRACTICAL PRESCRIPTION 9: THE LEAP

Now, I'm proud of you for making it all the way to this point. But I want to remind you it's not over yet. Just *reading* the book is not going to cut it. The idea is to ask the right, skillful questions *regularly*, and act on your instinct to find the best answers for yourself. I encourage you to now look at the whole of the slow medicine prescription—the 77 Skillful Questions list—which follows this chapter, and spend some time thinking about or writing down your intuitive answers. You might be inclined to feel this is a lot to do. Don't fret:

- Start by looking at the questions and working on just a few that seem *easy* to you. This will give you some traction and a sense of achievement, and help to clean up some low-hanging fruit. You'll be surprised at the considerable amount of energy this will give you, and the preparation will help you as you transition into potentially more difficult questions.
- Then go back to questions that might be challenging (but doable) and work on one or two of those at a time.
- Eventually, as you feel better (which you will), only then identify some core issues—the really challenging

questions—and develop a plan and a commitment to
finally tackle those.

Over time this method will help you to get through much of the
work. It might take months for you to address the "easy" questions;
the more challenging ones may take years. But if you stick to the plan,
you'll get there; and you'll feel better and better each step along the
way. In fact, you're likely to feel better *now*, just knowing you have a
plan that makes so much sense!

Don't let the herd knock you off course. It takes courage to go
in another direction given the influence of our modern society and
our susceptibility to the words of others. The path I have laid before
you is not new or unique. However, the message, as it is popularly
presented, has lost much of its essence and, therefore, its efficacy. The
work I am describing takes preparation. The next step is more like a
leap. Really, it's a genuine leap of faith, because we must break away
from the stronghold of those who would tell us that there is an easy
way to do this.

Before diving off a high cliff, it's best to make sure your final
step is square and balanced toward the water below, lest you go
tumbling over the rock face-first and *splat*. Slow medicine might
necessitate a plunge, but not a tumble. It's about working hard to
find and to move into your center, in integrity, square within yourself. It's about having a true, clear, and deep understanding of your
relationship to your body, mind, spirit, other people, the natural
world around you, and every aspect of the world. It's about alignment. That's the skillful path to peace and harmony, happiness, and
extraordinary health.

I have a very wise karate teacher who described the achievement
of becoming a black belt in this way: He said that some people think
that attaining the rank of black belt is the goal of the journey. In real-

ity, he said, it's just preparation to hike the mountain. When you get your black belt, it means that you've acquired some necessary skills and equipment—the physical endurance and the moves, the boots and the walking stick. In the process, you've inched closer to the mountain. Finally, you're there, but you're there at the foot of the mountain, not the top. It takes courage, humility, commitment—and hard work—to reach the summit.

Similarly, I set out to write this book with the goal of helping you develop the confidence in your *own* ability to find extraordinary health by learning to ask the right questions, and preparing you for the journey up the mountain. Now you have the right equipment and the right framework. The slow medicine prescription for success is natural, organic, simple, holistic, and utterly achievable. But it won't be easy. No journey to find treasure ever is. It will take some work, for sure. But now you know the most skillful way to get there. I wish you great success in your journey, and I'm honored that I could be the one to see you off. I hope to see you later on down the road.

77. What Are You Waiting For?

THE SLOW MEDICINE PRESCRIPTION:
77 SKILLFUL QUESTIONS FOR
EXTRAORDINARY HEALTH

A Review of All the Questions

1. What brings you here?
2. Are you free of all aches, pains, and chronic diseases?
3. Do you understand the causes of your chronic physical conditions?
4. Are you taking more medicines than you would like?
5. Do you feel a strong sense of purpose in life?
6. Do you believe it's possible to achieve genuine, extraordinary health?
7. Do you see an alignment between your personal and professional goals?
8. Does your job use all of your greatest talents, and is it enjoyable and fulfilling?
9. Are all your senses acute?
10. Do you take time to experience sensual pleasures in healthy ways?

11. Do you listen to your intuition?

12. Are you relaxed and in a calm state of mind when you eat?

13. Are the environments you live in clean, pure, and conducive to health and peace?

14. Are you grateful for the blessings in your life?

15. Do you feel physically attractive?

16. Do you think of and treat your body as a series of unrelated parts or a whole and unified system?

17. Are you conscious of the causes of your physical conditions and aware they might lie outside the body?

18. Do you take walks, garden, or have other regular contact with nature?

19. Do you feel energized or empowered by nature?

20. Do you engage in regular physical activity, and are you as physically strong as you'd like to be, with good endurance and aerobic capacity?

21. Do you fall asleep easily and soundly, and do you wake up feeling rested?

22. Do you observe a day of rest completely away from work, dedicated to nurturing yourself and your family?

23. Do you feel a strong connection to and appreciation for your home and your environment?

24. Do you take time to relax with activities that require abandon or absorption or play?

25. Do you maintain physically challenging goals?

26. Do you believe it's possible to change?

27. Are you happy with your body and at or near a healthy body weight?

28. Do you maintain a skillful diet, low in processed and refined foods and animal products and high in fresh, seasonal fruits and vegetables?

29. Is your water intake adequate?

30. Do you stretch regularly?

31. Have you let go of fear in your life?

32. Do you have faith in a god, spirit guides, angels, or some other power beyond yourself?

33. Do you actively commit time to your spiritual life?

34. Do you breathe abdominally for at least a few minutes a day?

35. Are you free from anger toward God?

36. Is the home you live in harmonious?

37. Do you have an awareness of life energy or chi?

38. Do you have more than enough energy to deal with your daily responsibilities?

39. Do you maintain peace of mind and tranquillity?

40. Can you reevaluate your financial "needs" so that you're not working so hard for things that aren't important?

41. Are creative activities a part of your work or leisure time?

42. Are you okay with a few surprises on your path to health?

43. Are you willing to take risks and make "mistakes" in order to succeed?

44. Are you able to adjust beliefs and attitudes as a result of learning from painful experiences, and has your experience of pain enabled you to grow spiritually?

45. Are you able to let go of your attachment to specific outcomes and embrace uncertainty?

46. Do you engage in meditation, contemplation, or psychotherapy to better understand your feelings?

47. Are you accepting of all your feelings?

48. Are you aware of and able to safely express sadness, anger, and fear, and do you have the ability to cry?

49. If you have experienced the loss of a loved one, have you fully grieved that loss?

50. Do you take risks or exceed previous limits?
51. Do you have the ability to concentrate for extended periods of time?
52. Is your sleep free from disturbing dreams, and do you explore the symbolism and emotional content of your dreams?
53. Are you free of any drug or alcohol dependency (including nicotine and caffeine)?
54. Did you or do you feel close with your parents?
55. Can you forgive yourself and others?
56. Do you enjoy high self-esteem?
57. Do you experience unconditional love?
58. Do you give yourself more supportive messages than critical messages?
59. Do you surround yourself with positive, encouraging people?
60. Do you experience intimate, nonsexual relationships?
61. Is your sexual relationship gratifying?
62. Do you feel a sense of belonging to a group or community?
63. Do you go out of your way to help others?
64. Do you confide in or speak openly with one or more close friends?
65. Have you demonstrated the willingness to commit to marriage or a comparable long-term relationship?
66. Have you had deep tissue bodywork or a massage, and are you comfortable being touched?
67. Can you let go of your self-interest in deciding the best course of action for a given situation?
68. Do you have regular, effortless bowel movements?
69. Have you conquered your fear of getting old and dying?
70. Are you willing to learn from children?

71. Do you actively pursue your goals and legacy, even as you age and suffer loss?

72. Do you experience feelings of joy and exhilaration?

73. Is your outlook basically optimistic, or can you envision yourself as more optimistic?

74. Are playfulness and humor important to you and do you have a sense of humor?

75. Do you feel a strong need to be right or in control?

76. Why do you have the symptoms you have now, and why these specific symptoms?

77. What are you waiting for?

ACKNOWLEDGMENTS

I Could Not Have Done This Alone

I WAS SEVEN WHEN I DECIDED to become a doctor. My father's mother was quite insistent on my fulfilling this dream, so it would make sense to start by acknowledging her influence. But, even before then, when I was just four, my mother had already noticed my "sensitivity," a particular way I had of soothing people with words and a kind hand: she predicted I would become a rabbi. She was not that far off, and she never let me forget how vital the heart and soul were in the practice of medicine that I would eventually study. But it was my children, Malcolm, Benjamin, and Caroline, who led me to where I am today, requiring that I fully integrate these elements of my nature and bridge the two disciplines. It was in my dedication to being a father that I learned to be a better person, and thus, a better doctor.

Along the way, many others steered me in the right direction, challenging and inspiring me with their wisdom and knowledge. Dr. Robert Ivker introduced me to holistic and integrative medicine, and became an early friend and influence. Indeed, his Wellness Self Test—

now known as the Fully Alive Questionnaire—was the foundation
for this book. My mentor and friend, Dr. Andrew Weil, whose passion created the Program in Integrative Medicine at the University of
Arizona (now known as the Arizona Center for Integrated Medicine),
provided me with an organized model on which to build my practice. My medical school classmate, Dr. Mehmet Oz, became the most
visible and voluble spokesperson for a more holistic understanding of
human health, opening many eyes to this work and creating more of
an audience than ever before.

But to write a book takes something well beyond the education
I received. It wasn't until I met David Nayor, who interviewed me
for a story on the medicinal value of yoga, that I heard someone say,
"I can help you write your message." Over four years, he picked my
brain and transcribed our conversations to prepare the earliest manuscript, which became the basis for the work I now call Skillful Living.
I am deeply indebted to David's patience and his abilities as a writer.
Equally important and essential, when I needed a new pair of eyes,
Ellen Daly appeared to help me refine the work, taking it to the next
level. It succeeded, and, with that, I found Celeste Fine, at Sterling
Lord Literistic, who masterfully agented this book into the capable
hands of Cassie Jones at William Morrow and Ian Blake Newhem,
a remarkably sensitive human being and writer extraordinaire, who
pulled everything together, helping me complete the manuscript and
bring it to its final form. In each, I found not only the skill I needed,
but individuals with passion for helping others. Along the way, my
family at Trent and Company, including my publicist, Nancy Trent,
and her capable team of Walter Sperr, Pam Wadler, Rachel Golden,
Angela Bonnici, Jen Homa, and Vida Engstrand, have treated me like
a brother as much as a client. And then there is my friend Loretta
Reilly, whose ability to create and capture images produced the illus-
trations for the book and the author photograph. This work is truly a

collaboration, and would not have been possible without all of these people.

In addition, my many friends, and my colleagues at SunRaven and in the Bedford community, continuously enrich my life and support my work. My sisters, Eve and Deborah, have been there always, and my father and mother have never suggested I return to being a conventional doctor and give up this dream of being something much more. I couldn't do this without their love.

But it's you, and all my patients like you, who actually provided me the stories and inspiration to refine my approach to health and healing. Clearly, the medical system needs improvement, and your demands for that motivated me to write this book.

There is nothing more important to our health than our relationships. In the end, I come back to this, and to the final acknowledgment of my muse, my dear and beloved, sweet, kind, and beautiful Robin, who challenges me more than any other, and has more capacity for forgiveness and growth than I have encountered in a partner ever before. Without the energy from this love, I would have no chance of achieving extraordinary health myself.

I am deeply grateful.

NOTES

EPIGRAPH

1. Moses Maimonides, "Physician's Prayer," *Congregation* Kol Ami *Shabbat Morning Prayer Book,* 3rd ed. (White Plains, NY: 1998).

INTRODUCTION

1. Dante Alighieri, "Inferno," in *The Portable Dante,* ed., trans., Mark Musa (New York: Penguin, 2003), 3.
2. Dr. Robert Ivker and Edward Zorensky, *Thriving: The Complete Mind/Body Guide for Optimal Health and Fitness for Men* (New York: Crown, 1997).
3. David M. Cutler, "The American Healthcare System," Harvard Essay Series: Healthcare Systems, last modified June 2008, http://www.medical.siemens.com/siemens/en_US/rg_marcom_FBAs/files/brochures/magazin_medicalsolutions_06_2008/MedSol_Jun_2008_e_Essay_Healthcare_System_USA.pdf.pdf.
4. "Americans' View on the Quality of Healthcare," Harvard School of Public Health and the Robert Wood Johnson Foundation, last modified March 18, 2011, http://www.hsph.harvard.edu/news/press-releases/poll-us-health-care-quality/.

CHAPTER 1

1. Andrew Taylor Still, *Philosophy of Osteopathy* (Kirksville, MO: A. T. Still, 1899), 28.

2. "Chronic Disease Prevention and Health Promotion," Centers for Disease Control and Prevention, last modified July 6, 2011, http://www.cdc.gov/chronicdisease/index.htm.

3. Jeffrey M. Jones, "Ratings of US Healthcare Quality, Coverage Best in 10 Years," Gallup, last modified November 19, 2010, accessed May 22, 2012, http://www.gallup.com/poll/144848/Ratings-Healthcare-Quality-Coverage-Best-Years.aspx.

4. Jonathan Cohn, *Sick: The Untold Story of America's Health Care Crisis—And the People Who Pay the Price* (New York: HarperCollins, 2007), 225.

5. "Successes and Opportunities for Population-Based Prevention and Control: At a Glance 2011," Centers for Disease Control and Prevention, last modified August 1, 2011, http://www.cdc.gov/chronicdisease/resources/publications/AAG/ddt.htm.

6. James O. Prochaska, John C. Norcross, and Carlo C. Diclemente, *Changing for Good: A Revolutionary Six-Stage Program for Overcoming Bad Habits and Moving Your Life Positively Forward* (New York: William Morrow, 2006), 62.

7. "Diabetes Basics," American Diabetes Association, accessed May 12, 2012, http://www.diabetes.org/diabetes-basics/type-1/.

8. Qiuping Gu, Charles F. Dillon, and Vicki L. Burt, "Prescription Drug Use Continues to Increase: US Prescription Drug Data for 2007–2008," National Center for Health Statistics, September 2010, http://www.cdc.gov/nchs/data/databriefs/db42.htm.

9. "Abilify (aripiprazole)," Abilify, accessed May 22, 2012, http://www.abilify.com.

10. "Fatal Combinations of Prescription Drugs," *Recovery Programs & Treatment Centers,* accessed May 22, 2012, http://www.recoverycorps.org/addiction/mixingdrugs/fatal-drug-combinations/.

11. John E. Sarno, *Mind Over Back Pain: A Radically New Approach to the Diagnosis and Treatment of Back Pain* (New York: Berkley, 1999), 50.

12. Martin Bashir and Deborah Apton, "Rick Warren and Purpose-Driven Strife," *ABC Nightline,* last modified June 22, 2007, http://abcnews.go.com/Nightline/story?id=2914953&page=1.

13. Associated Press, "Atlanta Hostage turning around 'sad, tough' life,"

msnbc.com, last modified March 15, 2005, http://www.nbcnews.com/id/7188576/.

14. Eckhart Tolle, *A New Earth: Awakening to Your Life's Purpose* (New York: Plume, 2006), 258.

15. Rick Foster, Greg Hicks, and Jen Seda, *Choosing Brilliant Health: 9 Choices That Redefine What It Takes to Create Lifelong Vitality and Well-Being* (New York: Penguin/Perigee, 2008), 92.

16. Ibid., 93.

17. K. Tanno et al., "Association of *Ikigai* as a Positive Psychological Factor with All-Cause-Specific Mortality Among Middle-Aged and Elderly Japanese People: Findings from the Japan Collaborative Cohort Study," *Journal of Psychosomatic Research* 67 (2009), 67–75; more studies cited in Martin E. P. Seligman, *Flourish: A Visionary New Understanding of Happiness and Well-Being* (New York: Free Press, 2011).

18. Martin Pinquart. "Creating and Maintaining Purpose in Life in Old Age: A Meta-Analysis," *Ageing International* 27, no. 2 (2002), 90.

19. Patricia Boyle, Aron S. Buchman, Lisa L. Barnes, and David A. Bennet, "Effect of a Purpose in Life on Risk of Incident Alzheimer's Disease and Mild Cognitive Impairment in Community-Dwelling Older Persons," *Archives of General Psychiatry* 67, no. 3 (2010), 304–10.

20. Ibid.

21. Sheldon Cohen, Cuneyt M. Alper, William J. Doyle, John J. Treanor, and Ronald B. Turner, "Positive Emotional Style Predicts Resistance to Illness After Experimental Exposure to Rhinovirus or Influenza A Virus," *Psychosomatic Medicine* 68, no. 6 (2006), 809–15.

22. Seligman, *Flourish*.

23. Ibid.

CHAPTER 2

1. Hippocrates, *Hippocrates, Volume 4*, trans. William Henry Samuel Jones (Cambridge, MA: Harvard University Press, 1967), 261.

2. T. Colin Campbell, *The China Study* (Dallas: BenBella Books, 2004), 76.

3. Centers for Disease Control and Prevention, *National Diabetes Fact Sheet: General Information and National Estimates on Diabetes in the United States, 2005* (Atlanta, GA: Department of Health and Human Services, 2005).

4. Brian Wansink, *Mindless Eating* (New York: Bantam Dell, 2006).

5. Ezra Pound, "In a Station of the Metro," in *Lustra* (New York: Alfred A. Knopf, 1917), 50.

6. Ralph Waldo Emerson, "Self-Reliance," in *Nature and Selected Essays* (London: Penguin Classics, 2003), 176.

7. Annette Prüss-Üstün and Carlos F. Corvalán, "Preventing disease through healthy environments—towards an estimate of the environmental burden of disease," World Health Organization, 2006.

8. Ibid.

9. E. C. Matsui et al., "Asthma in the Inner City and the Indoor Environment," *Immunology and Allergy Clinics of North America* 28, no. 3 (2008), 665–86.

10. "A–Z of Environmental Health," National Institute of Environmental Health Science, National Institutes of Health, accessed May 22, 2012, http://www.niehs.nih.gov/health/topics/atoz/.

CHAPTER 3

1. William Wordsworth, "Lines Composed a Few Miles Above Tintern Abbey," in *Lyrical Ballads, with a Few Other Poems* (London: J. & A. Arch, 1798), 207.

2. Albert Ellis and Robert A. Harper, *A Guide to Rational Living* (Chatsworth, CA: Wilshire Book Company–Melvin Powers, 1975), 174.

3. Richard Louv, *Last Child in the Woods: Saving Our Children from Nature-Deficit Disorder* (North Carolina: Algonquin, 2008), 36.

4. "Summary of Findings, Sleep in America Poll," National Sleep Foundation, March 2, 2009, http://www.sleepfoundation.org/sites/default/files/2009%20Sleep%20in%20America%20SOF%20EMBARGOED.pdf.

5. "Sleep Disorders," National Institute of Neurological Disorders and Stroke, National Institutes of Health, last modified May 21, 2007, http://www.ninds.nih.gov/disorders/brain_basics/understanding_sleep.htm#sleep_disorders.

6. Steven Reinberg, "Millions of Americans Don't Get Enough Sleep," *US News and World Report,* October 29, 2009, accessed May 22, 2012, http://health.usnews.com/health-news/family-health/sleep/articles/2009/10/29/millions-of-americans-dont-get-enough-sleep.

7. "Short Sleep Duration Among Workers—United States, 2010," Center for Disease Control and Prevention, April 27, 2012, http://www.cdc.gov/mmwr/pdf/wk/mm6116.pdf.

8. "America's Huge Sleep Deficit," *The Week,* May 18, 2012, 21.

9. "U.S. Sleep Aids Market Now Worth $23 Billion as Americans Battle Insomnia, Sleep Disorders," *Marketdata Enterprises,* June 2008, 1–3.

10. Tim Arnott, *Dr. Arnott's 24 Realistic Ways to Improve Your Health* (Nampa, ID: Pacific Press, 2004), 2.

11. M. L. Perlis et al., "Insomnia as a risk factor for onset of depression in the elderly," *Behavioral Sleep Medicine* 4, no. 2 (2006), 104–13.

12. D. Riemann and U. Voderholzer, "Primary insomnia: a risk factor to develop depression?" *Journal of Affective Disorders* 76, nos. 1–3 (2003), 255–59.

13. Franklin House, Stuart A. Seale, and Ian Blake Newman, *The 30-Day Diabetes Miracle* (New York: Penguin/Perigee, 2008), 248–49.

14. M. Beckett and L. C. Roden, "Mechanisms by which circadian rhythm disruption may lead to cancer," *South African Journal of Science* 105 (2009), 415.

15. "Sleep and Sleep Disorders," Centers for Disease Control and Prevention, last modified March 1, 2012, http://www.cdc.gov/sleep/.

16. Andrew Weil, *8 Weeks to Optimum Health* (New York: Knopf, 1997), 101.

17. Lao Tzu, "Thoughts from the Tao Te Ching," in *A World of Ideas,* 8th ed., ed. Lee A. Jacobus (New York: Bedford/St. Martin's, 2009).

18. Centers for Disease Control and Prevention, *Fertility, Family Planning, and Reproductive Health of U.S. Women: Data from the 2002 National Survey of Family Growth* (Atlanta, GA: Department of Health and Human Services, 2005).

19. Christiane Northrup, *Women's Bodies, Women's Wisdom* (New York: Bantam, 2010), 114.

CHAPTER 4

1. Portia Nelson, *There's a Hole in My Sidewalk: The Romance of Self-Discovery* (New York: Atria Books/Beyond Words, 2012), xi–xii.

2. Nick Dowling and Gary Luffman, "The Application of Neuroscience in L&D and Change Management," Association of Business Psychologists, accessed May 22, 2012, http://theabp.org.uk/images/uploads/Blue_Edge-Neuroscience_in_LD-ABP2012.pdf.

3. Martin E. P. Seligman, *Helplessness: On Depression, Development, and Death* (San Francisco: Freeman, 1975).

4. Madelon A. Visintainer, Joseph R. Volpicelli, and Martin E. P. Seligman,

"Tumor Rejection in Rats After Inescapable or Escapable Shock," *Science* 216, no. 4544 (1982), 437–39.

5. J. Bruce Overmier, "On learned helplessness," *Integrative Physiological and Behavioral Science* 37, no. 1 (2002), 4–8.

6. W. C. Miller, "How effective are traditional dietary and exercise interventions for weight loss?" *Medicine and Science in Sports and Exercise* 31, no. 8 (1999), 1129–34.

7. Thich Thien-An, *Zen Philosophy, Zen Practice* (Berkeley, CA: Dharma, 1975), 73.

8. Gustave Le Bon, *The Crowd: A Study of the Popular Mind* (New York: Macmillan, 1896), 171; http://etext.virginia.edu/toc/modeng/public/BonCrow.html.

9. W. D. Hamilton, "Geometry for the Selfish Herd," *Journal of Theoretical Biology* 31 (1971), 295–311.

10. Lauren F. Friedman, "Rabble with a Cause: Were the London Riots a Spontaneous Mass Reaction or a Rational Response?" *Scientific American*, last updated August 12, 2011, http://www.scientificamerican.com/article .cfm?id=rabble-with-a-cause.

11. Louis René Beres, "Dangers of the Herd Mentality," *Washington Times,* last updated February 27, 2006, accessed June 21, 2012, http://www.washing tontimes.com/news/2006/feb/27/20060227-093416-9462r/.

12. Jim Nuovo, ed., *Chronic Disease Management* (New York: Springer, 2007), 327.

13. Brenda Davis and Vasanto Melina, *Becoming Vegan: The Complete Guide to Adopting a Healthy Plant-Based Diet* (Summertown, TN: Book Publishing, 2000), 206.

14. Lester R. Brown et al., *State of the World 2000* (New York: W. W. Norton and Company, 2000), xviiii.

15. Franklin House, Stuart A. Seale, and Ian Blake Newman. *The 30-Day Diabetes Miracle* (New York: Penguin/Perigee, 2008), xi.

16. "Profiling Food Consumption in America," *Agricultural Fact Book,* United States Department of Agriculture, last modified 2002, http://www.usda .gov/wps/portal/usda/usdahome?contentid=agfactbook.xml&navid=AG_ FACT_BOOK.

17. "Portion Distortion: Serving Sizes Are Growing," *Meals Matter,* http://

www.mealsmatter.org/articles-and-resources/healthy-living-articles/ Portion-Distortion.aspx.

18. T. Colin Campbell, *The China Study* (Dallas: BenBella Books, 2006), 141.

19. Associated Press, "Patients lie to doctors—and suffer for it," msnbc .com, last modified February 16, 2007, http://www.msnbc.msn.com/ id/17188153/ns/health-health_care/t/patients-lie-doctors-suffer-it/.

20. Jon Kabat-Zinn, "Psychosocial Factors in Coronary Heart Disease: Their Importance and Management," quoted in *Prevention of Coronary Heart Disease*, eds., I. S. Ockene, and J. Ockene (Boston: Little, Brown, 1993), 299–333.

21. "Water: How Much Should You Drink Every Day?" Mayo Clinic, last updated October 12, 2011, accessed May 1, 2012, http://www.mayoclinic .com/health/water/NU00283.

22. Bob Anderson, *Stretching* (Bolinas, CA: Shelter Publications, 2000), 11.

23. "How Much Information? 2009 Report on American Consumers," Global Information Industry Center, last modified January, 2010, http://hmi .ucsd.edu/howmuchinfo_research_report_consum.php.

24. David French, *Everything Is Bad for You: An A–Z Guide to What You Never Knew Could Kill You* (Naperville, IL: Sourcebooks Hysteria, 2002).

25. Financial Times and Harris Interactive, "Religious Views and Beliefs Vary Greatly by Country, According to the Latest Financial Times/Harris Poll," last modified December 20, 2006, accessed September 4, 2011, http://www.harrisinteractive.com/NEWS/allnewsbydate .asp?NewsID=1130.

26. G. Gallup, *Religion in America: 1990* (Princeton, NJ: Princeton Religious Research Center, 1985).

27. D. A. Matthews, Michael E. McCullough, and David B. Larson, "Religious Commitment and Health Status: A Review of the Research and Implications for Family Medicine," *Archives of Family Medicine* 7, no. 2 (1998), 118–24.

28. Harold G. Koenig, Michael E. McCullough, and David B. Larson, *Handbook of Religion and Health* (New York: Oxford University Press, 2001), 7–14.

29. George W. Comstock and Kay B. Partridge, "Church Attendance and Health," *Journal of Chronic Diseases* 25, no. 12 (1965), 665–72.

30. Jeff Levin, *God, Faith, and Healing: Exploring the Spirituality and Healing Connection* (New York: Wiley, 2001), 55.

31. Randolph C. Byrd, "Positive Therapeutic Effects of Intercessory Prayer in a Coronary Care Unit Population," *Southern Medical Journal* 81, no. 7 (1988), 826–29.

32. Harold G. Koenig, "Religion, Spirituality, and Medicine: Application to Clinical Practice," *Journal of the American Medical Association* 4 (2000), 1708.

33. Xu Jianbin, and Kalyani K. Mehta, "The Effects of Religion on Subjective Aging in Singapore: An Interreligious Comparison," *Journal of Aging Studies* 17 (2003): 485–502.

34. Ibid.

35. Ibid.

36. William James, "What Is an Emotion?" *Mind* 9, no. 34 (1884): 188–205.

CHAPTER 5

1. Ronald W. Clark, *Einstein: The Life and Times* (New York: Avon, 2001), 422.

2. Thich Nhat Hanh, *The Sun My Heart* (Berkeley, CA: Parallax Press, 1988), 32, 79.

3. "Resources," United Indians of All Tribes Foundation, accessed May 22, 2012, http://www.unitedindians.org/resources001.html.

4. Reverend Martin Luther King Jr., "The American Dream," in *A Testament of Hope: The Essential Writings and Speeches of Martin Luther King, Jr.*, ed. James M. Washington (New York: HarperOne, 1991), 210.

5. Lao Tzu, "Negotiating *Te*," in *Tao Te Ching: The Way of Virtue*, trans. Patrick Byrne (New York: Square One Publishers, 2001), 45.

6. Henry David Thoreau, *Walden; Or, Life in the Woods* (New York: Dover, 1995), 53.

7. Stephen R. Covey, *The 7 Habits of Highly Effective People* (New York: Free Press, 1989).

8. Joseph Campbell and Bill Moyers, *The Power of Myth* (Maine: Anchor, 1991), 113.

9. James Joyce, *Ulysses* (New York: Vintage, 1990), 190.

10. "The Legend of the Cracked Pot," quoted in Sam Louie, *Asian Honor: Overcoming the Culture of Silence* (Bloomington, IN: WestBow Press, 2012), 101.

CHAPTER 6

1. Carl G. Jung, *The Earth Has a Soul: C.G. Jung on Nature, Technology & Modern Life*, ed. Meredith Sabini (Berkeley, CA: North Atlantic Books, 2011), 59.

2. William Faulkner, "A Rose for Emily," *Selected Short Stories of William Faulkner* (New York: Modern Library, 2012), 52.

3. Joshua D. Foster and Ilan Shrira, "The Occupation with the Highest Suicide Rate," *Psychology Today,* last updated August 1, 2009, accessed June 21, 2012, http://www.psychologytoday.com/blog/the-narcissus-in-all-us/200908/the-occupation-the-highest-suicide-rate.

4. David Noonan, "Doctors Who Kill Themselves," *Newsweek,* last updated April 19, 2008, http://www.newsweek.com/2008/04/19/doctors-who-kill-themselves.html.

5. Thich Nhat Hanh, *Anger: Wisdom for Cooling the Flames* (New York: Riverhead Books, 2002), 77.

6. Benedict Carey, "Grief Could Join List of Disorders," *New York Times*, last modified January 24, 2012, accessed May 30, 2012, http://www.nytimes.com/2012/01/25/health/depressions-criteria-may-be-changed-to-include-grieving.html.

7. Allen Frances, "Don't Confuse Grief with Depression," *Huffington Post*, last modified January 27, 2012, accessed May 30, 2012, http://www.huffingtonpost.com/allen-frances/dont-confuse-grief-with-d_b_1233883.html.

8. Leeat Granek et al., "Nature and Impact of Grief Over Patient Loss on Oncologists' Personal and Professional Lives," *Archives of Internal Medicine* 172, no. 12 (2012), 964–96.

9. Leeat Granek, "When Doctors Grieve," *New York Times*, last modified March 25, 2012, accessed May 30, 2012, http://www.nytimes.com/2012/05/27/opinion/sunday/when-doctors-grieve.html.

10. Granek, "Nature and Impact of Grief Over Patient Loss on Oncologists' Personal and Professional Lives."

11. Avery Corman, "Moving Through Grief, Chair by Chair," *New York Times*, last modified March 15, 2012, accessed May 30, 2012, http://www.nytimes.com/2012/03/18/fashion/moving-through-grief-chair-by-chair-modern-love.html.

12. Rick Foster, Greg Hicks, and Jen Seda, *Choosing Brilliant Health: 9 Choices*

That Redefine What It Takes to Create Lifelong Vitality and Well-Being (New York: Penguin, 2008), 111–34.

13. Ibid., 113.

14. John Powers, *Introduction to Tibetan Buddhism,* rev. ed. (Ithaca, NY: Snow Lion Publications, 2007), 326–27.

15. Sogyal Rinpoche, *The Tibetan Book of Living and Dying,* rev. ed. (New York: HarperOne, 2002), 8.

16. James Prochaska, John C. Norcross, and Carlo DiClemente, *Changing for Good: A Revolutionary Six-Stage Program for Overcoming Bad Habits and Moving Your Life Positively Forward* (New York: William Morrow, 2006), 15.

17. Adapted from ibid., 39–46.

18. Shamsi T. Iqbal and Eric Horvitz, "Disruption and Recovery of Computing Tasks: Field Study, Analysis, and Directions," Microsoft, last updated March 2007, accessed May 30, 2012, http://research.microsoft.com/en-us/um/people/horvitz/CHI_2007_Iqbal_Horvitz.pdf.

19. Paul E. Dux, Jason Ivanoff, Christopher L. Asplund, and René Marois, "Isolation of a Central Bottleneck of Information Processing with Time-Resolved fMRI," *Neuron* 52, no. 6 (2006), 1109–20.

20. Jonathan B. Spira and Joshua B. Feintuch, "The Cost of Not Paying: How Interruptions Impact Knowledge Worker Productivity," Basex, accessed May 30, 2012, http://www.basex.com/web/tbghome.nsf/23e5e39594c06 4ee852564ae004fa010/ea4eae828bd411be8525742f0006cde3/$file/costof notpayingattention.basexreport.pdf.

21. Ibid.

22. Guilherme Polanczyk et al., "The Worldwide Prevalence of ADHD: A Systematic Review and Metaregression Analysis," *American Journal of Psychiatry* 164 (2007), 942–48.

23. L. Alan Sroufe, "Ritalin Gone Wrong," *New York Times,* last updated January 28, 2012, accessed May 30, 2012, http://www.nytimes.com/2012/01/29/opinion/sunday/childrens-add-drugs-dont-work-long-term.html.

24. Edward M. Hallowell, "Overloaded Circuits: Why Smart People Underperform," *Harvard Business Review,* January 2005, accessed May 30, 2012, http://www.integrity-plus.com/eStore/WP/overload%20cir cuitsR0501Ef2.pdf.

25. William John Ickes, Robert A. Wicklund, and C. Brian Ferris, "Objective

self awareness and self esteem," *Journal of Experimental Social Psychology* 9, no. 3 (1973), 202–19.

26. Joel Brockner and A. J. Blethyn Hulton, "How to reverse the vicious cycle of low self-esteem: The importance of attentional focus," *Journal of Experimental Social Psychology* 14, no. 6 (1978), 564–78.

CHAPTER 7

1. Anthony Robbins, in QuotationsBook, accessed June 21, 2012, http://quotationsbook.com/quotes/author/6152/page=2/.

2. Mahatma Gandhi and Richard Attenborough, *The Words of Gandhi,* 2nd ed. (New York: New Market Press, 2008), 55.

3. Helen Cheng and Adrian Furnham, "Personality, self-esteem, and demographic predictions of happiness and depression," *Personality and Individual Differences* 34, no. 6 (2003), 921–42.

4. Ibid.

5. Michael Marmot, "Self Esteem and Health," *British Medical Journal* 327 (2003), 574–75.

6. David Mills, afterword to Albert Ellis, "Overcoming 'Self-Esteem,'" Albert Ellis Institute, last modified 2003, accessed May 31, 2012, http://www.davidmills.net/index_files/Overcoming-Self-Esteem.pdf.

7. Ibid.

8. Ibid.

9. Ibid.

10. Norman Vincent Peale, *Positive Thinking for a Time Like This* (Upper Saddle River, NJ: Prentice-Hall, 1975), 62.

11. Martin E. P. Seligman, *Flourish: A Visionary New Understanding of Happiness and Well-being* (New York: Free Press, 2012).

12. Harville Hendrix, *Getting the Love You Want: A Guide for Couples: 20th Anniversary Edition* (New York: Henry Holt and Company, 2008), 85–90.

13. Roberto De Vogli, Tarani Chandola, and Michael Gideon Marmot, "Negative Aspects of Close Relationships and Heart Disease," *Archive of Internal Medicine* 167, no. 18 (2007), 1951–57.

14. Karen J. Prager, *The Psychology of Intimacy* (New York: The Guilford Press, 1995), 1.

15. Ibid., 2

16. Ute Schulz and Ralf Schwarzer, "Long-term Effects of Spousal Support on

Coping with Cancer After Surgery," *Journal of Social and Clinical Psychology* 23, no. 5 (2004), 716–32.

17. Stevan E. Hobfoll and Arie Nadler, "Satisfaction with Social Support During Crisis: Intimacy and Self-Esteem as Critical Determinants," *Journal of Personality and Social Psychology* 51, no. 2 (1986), 296-304.

18. Carol D. Ryff and Corey Lee M. Keyes, "The Structure of Psychological Well-Being Revisited," *Journal of Personality and Social Psychology* 69, no. 4 (1995), 719–27.

19. Robert A. Emmons, "Personal goals, life meaning, and virtue: Wellsprings of a positive life," quoted in *Flourishing: Positive Psychology and the Life Well-Lived*, eds. Corey Lee M. Keyes and Jonathan Haidt (Washington: American Psychological Association, 2003), 105–28.

20. Ibid.

21. Dan P. McAdams and Fred B. Bryant, "Intimacy Motivation and Subjective Mental Health in a Nationwide Sample," *Journal of Personality* 55, no. 3 (1987), 395–413.

22. Ibid.

23. David M. Harvey, Cynthia J. Curry, and James H. Bray, "Individuation and Intimacy in Intergenerational Relationships and Health: Patterns Across Two Generations," *Journal of Family Psychology* 5, no. 2 (1991), 204–36.

24. Henri J. M. Nouwen, *Bread for the Journey: A Daybook of Wisdom and Faith* (New York: HarperOne, 1996), 55.

25. Elizabeth Lesser, *Broken Open: How Difficult Times Can Help Us Grow* (New York: Villard Books, 2005).

26. Kahlil Gibran, *The Prophet* (Hertfordshire, UK: Wordsworth Editions Limited, 1996), 7.

27. Marcel Proust, "Ephemeral Efficacy of Grief," *The Complete Short Stories of Marcel Proust,* trans. Joachim Neugroschel (Lanham, MD: Cooper Square Press, 2001), 125.

28. David Wolpe, "Space in Togetherness," Sinai Temple, last updated May 11, 2012, accessed June 21, 2012, http://sinaitemple.org/learning_with_ the_rabbis/writings/2012/051012SpacesInTogetherness.pdf.

29. Martin Buber, *I and Thou* (London, UK: Continuum, 2004), 51.

30. Wolpe, "Space in Togetherness."

31. Robert Brault, "Final Thoughts for 2011," last updated December 21,

2011, accessed June 11, 2012, http://www.robertbrault.com/2011_12_01_
archive.html.

32. Rory Freedman and Kim Barnouin, *Skinny Bitch* (Philadelphia: Running Press, 2005), 117.

33. Keith N. Hampton, Lauren Sessions Goulet, Cameron Marlow, and Lee Rainie, "Why most Facebook users get more than they give," Pew Internet & American Life Project/Pew Research Center, last updated February 3, 2012, accessed June 2, 2012, http://www.pewinternet.org/~/media/Files/Reports/2012/PIP_Facebook%20users_2.3.12.pdf.

34. Randall Stross, "Social Networks, Small and Smaller," *New York Times,* last updated April 14, 2012, accessed June 2, 2012, http://www.nytimes.com/2012/04/15/business/path-familyleaf-and-pair-small-by-design-social-networks.html.

35. Aleks Krotoski, "Robin Dunbar: we can only ever have 150 friends at most . . ." *The Observer,* last updated March 13, 2010, accessed June 2, 2012, http://www.guardian.co.uk/technology/2010/mar/14/my-bright-idea-robin-dunbar.

36. Barack Obama, "National Volunteer Week, 2011: A Proclamation by the President of the United States of America," last updated April 7, 2011, accessed June 7, 2012, http://www.whitehouse.gov/the-press-office/2011/04/07/presidential-proclamation-national-volunteer-week.

37. Ibid.

38. C. Daniel Batson, *The Altruism Question: Toward a Social-Psychological Answer* (Hillsdale, NJ: Lawrence Erlbaum Associates, 1991), 6.

39. Martin L. Hoffman, "Psychological and Biological Perspectives on Altruism," *International Journal of Behavioral Development* 1 (1978), 323–39.

40. Larry Scherwitz et al., "Type A Behavior, Self-Involvement, and Coronary Atherosclerosis," *Psychosomatic Medicine* 45, no. 1 (1983), 47–57.

41. Michael Gurven, "The Evolution of Contingent Cooperation," *Current Anthropology* 47, no. 1 (2006), 185–92.

42. H. Kern Reeve and Bert Hölldobler, "The Emergence of a Superorganism through Intergroup Competition," *Proceedings of the National Academy of Sciences* 104, no. 23 (2007), 9736–40.

43. Adrian V. Bell, Peter J. Richerson, and Richard McElreath, "Culture Rather Than Genes Provides Greater Scope for the Evolution of Large-

Scale Human Prosociality," *Proceedings of the National Academy of Sciences* 106, no. 42 (2009), 17671–74.

44. Sang-Jin Ma, "Factors Influencing Productive Activities of the Korean Rural Elderly," *Journal of Rural Development* 31, no. 2 (2008), 23–35

45. Paul Arnstein et al., "From Chronic Pain Patient to Peer: Benefits and Risks of Volunteering," *Pain Management Nursing* 3, no. 3 (2002), 94–103.

46. Stephen G. Post, "Altruism, Happiness, and Health: It's Good to Be Good," *International Journal of Behavioral Medicine* 12, no. 2 (2005), 66–77.

47. David C. McClelland and Carol Kirshnit, "The Effect of Motivational Arousal Through Films on Salivary Immunoglobulin A," *Psychology and Health* 2, no. 1 (1988), 31–52.

48. Christine L. Carter, "What We Get When We Give," *Psychology Today,* last updated February 18, 2010, accessed June 4, 2012, http://www.psy chologytoday.com/blog/raising-happiness/201002/what-we-get-when-we-give.

49. Marc A. Musick, A. Regula Herzog, and James S. House, "Volunteering and Mortality among Older Adults: Findings from a National Sample," *Journals of Gerontology Series B: Psychological Sciences & Social Sciences* 54B, no. 3 (1999), S173–S180.

50. William Michael Brown, Nathan S. Consedine, and Carol Magai, "Altruism Relates to Health in an Ethnically Diverse Sample of Older Adults," *Journal of Gerontology: Psychological Sciences* 60B, no. 3 (2005), P143–P152.

51. Sara Konrath, Andrea Fuhrel-Forbis, Alina Lou, and Stephanie Brown, "Motives for Volunteering Are Associated with Mortality Risk in Older Adults," *Health Psychology* 31, no. 1 (2012), 87–96.

52. Michele Dillon, "Is It Good to Do Good? Altruism and Health," in *Taking Care of Self and Community: A University Dialogue on Health 2009–2010,* University of New Hampshire Discovery Program, last updated 2009, accessed June 4, 2012, http://scholars.unh.edu/discovery_ud/48.

53. Karen Allen, Barbara E. Shykoff, and Joseph L. Izzo Jr., "Pet Ownership, But Not ACE Inhibitor Therapy, Blunts Home Blood Pressure Responses to Mental Stress," *Hypertension* 38 (2001), 815–20.

54. Karen Allen, Jim Blascovich, and Wendy B. Mendes, "Cardiovascular Reactivity and the Presence of Pets, Friends, and Spouses: The Truth About Cats and Dogs," *Psychosomatic Medicine* 64, no. 5 (2002), 727–39.

55. State University of New York, Rockland, "Retired and Senior Volunteer

Program (RSVP): Statement of Values," accessed June 7, 2012, http://www.sunyrockland.edu/community/seniors/rsvps.

56. Tara Parker-Pope, "What Are Friends For? A Longer Life," *New York Times,* last updated April 20, 2009, accessed June 2, 2012, http://www.nytimes.com/2009/04/21/health/21well.html.

57. Annika Rosengren, Lars Wilhelmsen, and Kristina Orth-Gomér, "Coronary Disease in Relation to Social Support and Social Class in Swedish Men: A 15 Year Follow-Up in the Study of Men Born in 1933," *European Heart Journal* 25, no. 1 (2004), 56–63.

58. Kristina Orth-Gomér, Annika Rosengren, and Lars Wilhelmsen, "Lack of Social Support and Incidence of Coronary Heart Disease in Middle-Aged Swedish Men," *Psychosomatic Medicine* 55 (1993), 37–43.

59. Candyce H. Kroenke et al., "Social Networks, Social Support, and Survival After Breast Cancer Diagnosis," *Journal of Clinical Oncology* 24, no. 7 (2006), 1105–11.

60. Nicholas A. Christakis and James H. Fowler, "The Spread of Obesity in a Large Social Network over 32 Years," *New England Journal of Medicine* 357 (2007), 370–79.

CHAPTER 8

1. Mary Oliver, *New and Selected Poems, Volume One* (Boston: Beacon Press, 2004), 10–11.

2. Sam Martin, *How to Achieve Total Enlightenment: A Practical Guide to the Meaning of Life* (Kansas City, MO: Andrews McMeel Publishing, 2005), 101.

3. Steven R. Covey, *The 7 Habits of Highly Effective People* (New York: Free Press, 2004), 296.

4. David Leon Moore, "Many boomers race to keep fit, put focus on staying in shape," *USA Today,* last modified January 17, 2011, accessed June 13, 2012, http://www.usatoday.com/sports/2011-01-16-baby-boomers-athletes-marathon_N.htm.

5. Ronnie Crocker, "Boomers have high expectations for retirement," *Houston Chronicle,* last modified July 13, 2011, http://www.chron.com/business/article/Boomers-have-high-expectations-for-retirement-2078260.php.

6. Helen Rippier Wheeler, "Senior Power: Keirō no hi," *Berkeley Daily Planet,* last modified August 16, 2011, accessed June 13, 2012, http://www.berke

leydailyplanet.com/issue/2011-08-17/article/38250?headline=-Senior-Power-Keir-no-hi---By-Helen-Rippier-Wheeler.

7. Akiko Hashimoto, *The Gift of Generations: Japanese and American Perspectives on Aging and the Social Contract* (Cambridge: Cambridge University Press, 1996), 5.

8. James J. Dowd, "Aging and the Course of Desire," *Journal of Aging Studies* 26 (2012), 285–95.

9. Ibid.

10. Nancy Stein, Susan Folkman, Tom Trabasso, and T. Anne Richards, "Appraisal and Goal Processes as Predictors of Psychological Well-Being in Bereaved Caregivers," *Journal of Personality and Social Psychology* 72, no. 4 (1997), 872–84.

11. Ethel Shanas, "Aging and Life Space in Poland and the United States," *Journal of Health and Social Behavior* 11, no. 3 (1970), 183–90.

12. Melonie Heron, "Deaths: Leading Causes for 2008," *Centers for Disease Control and Prevention/National Vital Statistics Reports,* last modified June 6, 2012, accessed June 13, 2012, http://www.cdc.gov/nchs/data/nvsr/nvsr60/nvsr60_06.pdf.

13. Cheryl J. Hansen, Larry C. Stevens, and J. Richard Coast, "Exercise Duration and Mood State: How Much Is Enough to Feel Better?" *Health Psychology* 20, no. 4 (2001), 267–75.

14. David Leon Moore, "Many boomers race to keep fit, put focus on staying in shape," *USA Today,* last modified January 17, 2011, accessed June 13, 2012, http://www.usatoday.com/sports/2011-01-16-baby-boomers-athletes-marathon_N.htm.

15. Murray Drummond and James Smith, "Ageing Men's Understanding of Nutrition: Implications for Health," *Journal of Men's Health & Gender* 3, no. 1 (2006), 56–60.

16. Jiayin Liang and Baozhen Luo, "Toward a Discourse Shift in Social Gerontology: From Successful Aging to Harmonious Aging," *Journal of Aging Studies* 26, no. 3 (2012), 327–34.

17. James J. Dowd, "Aging and the Course of Desire," *Journal of Aging Studies* 26 (2012), 285–95.

18. Chau-kiu Cheung and Ping Kwong Kam, "Resiliency in Older Hong Kong Chinese: Using the Grounded Theory Approach to Reveal Social

and Spiritual Conditions," *Journal of Aging Studies* 26, no. 3 (2012), 355–67.

19. Bienke M. Janssen, Tineke A. Abma, and Tine Van Regenmortel, "Maintaining Mastery Despite Age Related Losses: The Resilience Narratives of Two Older Women in Need of Long-Term Community Care," *Journal of Aging Studies* 26, no. 3 (2012), 343–54.

20. Bob Kelly, *Worth Repeating: More Than 5,000 Classic and Contemporary Quotes* (Grand Rapids, MI: Kregel Academic & Professional, 2003), 98.

21. Barbara L. Fredrickson, "Cultivating Positive Emotions to Optimize Health and Well-Being," *Prevention & Treatment* 3 (2000), http://www.rickhanson.net/wp-content/files/papers/CultPosEmot.pdf.

22. Ibid.

23. Norman B. Anderson, *Emotional Longevity: What REALLY Determines How Long You Live* (New York: Viking, 2003), 243.

24. Stephen G. Post "Altruism, Happiness, and Health: It's Good to Be Good," *International Journal of Behavioral Medicine* 12 (2005), 66–77.

25. Ruut Veenhoven, "Healthy Happiness: Effects of happiness on physical health and the consequences for preventive health care," *Journal of Happiness Studies* 9 (2008), 449–69.

26. Fredrickson, "Cultivating Positive Emotions to Optimize Health and Well-Being."

27. David M. W. de Coverley Veale, "Exercise and mental health," *Acta Psychiatrica Scandinavica* 76 (1987), 113–20.

28. Chad M. Burton and Laura A. King, "The health benefits of writing about intensely positive experiences," *Journal of Research in Personality* 38, no. 2 (2004), 150–63.

29. Dick Prouty, Jane Paninucci, and Rufus Collinson, eds., *Adventure Education: Theory and Applications* (Champaign, IL: Human Kinetics, 2007), 69.

30. Erica Wilson and Donna E. Little, "Adventure and the gender gap: acknowledging diversity of experience," *Loisir et Societé/Society & Leisure* 28, no. 1 (2005), 185–208.

31. Pat Rodegast and Judith Stanton, *Emmanuel's Book: A Manual for Living Comfortably in the Cosmos* (New York: Bantam, 1987), 3.

32. James Baldwin, *The Cross of Redemption: Uncollected Writings* (New York: Vintage, 2011), 42.

CHAPTER 9

1. Albert Einstein and Leopold Infeld, *The Evolution of Physics* (New York: Touchstone, 1967), 152.

2. David Joseph Schwartz, *The Magic of Thinking Big* (New York: Fireside, 2007), 51.

INDEX

A-game, medical, 12–14, 51
abuse, 227, 228, 230, 249, 262
acceptance: belonging and, 253; of
  death, 208–9, 279–80; of family,
  227–31; Medicine Wheel and, 7;
  self-, 234–40
acupuncture, 117, 202
addictions. *See* substance abuse
"adventure education," 291
Agency for Research on Cancer, 105
aging: action cures for, 280–83;
  anti-279, 280–82; change and,
  287; definition of skillful, 286; as
  disease state, 281; fear of, 212–14,
  265–76, 279, 280–83; Japanese
  culture and, 282–83; "New Old,"
  282; as normal, 281; positive
  emotions and, 288–91; purpose in
  life and, 283; pursuit of goals and
  legacy and, 283–88; quality of life
  and, 285; relationships and, 281;
  resiliency and, 287
alcohol, 29, 103. *See also* substance
  abuse
aloneness, 151, 153, 205
altruism, 255–57
American Board of Integrative
  Holistic Medicine, 11
American Psychiatric Association,
  208
Anderson, Norman B., 289
anger: concentration/focusing and,
  220; eating and, 137; expressing
  and managing, 201, 203–4,
  205–7; Finkelstein transition and,
  197; getting unstuck and, 176;

holding on to, 162; Karen's case
  and, 201, 203–4; liver as organ
  associated with, 271; mind-body
  connection and, 304; as negative
  emotion, 289; positive feelings
  and, 290; questions about, 12, 160;
  relationships and, 227, 229, 246;
  sharing of, 203; Steven's case and,
  271, 272, 273, 274
animal products: anti-inflammatory
  lifestyle and, 29; questions about,
  134–43
anxiety: ADD and, 220; belonging
  and, 256; change and, 189, 216;
  concentration/focusing and, 220;
  about death, 212; denial and,
  142; eating and, 137; expressing,
  205; and fear of death, 214;
  forgiveness and, 233; guided
  imagery and, 221; information
  overload and, 149; learning from
  children and, 277; materialism
  and, 60; as negative emotion,
  289; relationships and, 245, 247;
  self-esteem and, 236; senses and,
  63; about sex, 248; universality of,
  220. *See also* fear
appreciation. *See* gratitude
Aristotle, 203
attachment, 190–93, 197, 212,
  227, 241, 242, 280, 302. *See also*
  connections
attention deficit disorder (ADD/
  ADHD), 95, 219–20
authenticity, 7, 36, 63, 214
Avatamsaka Sutra, 166